burn

burn

THE BURN BOOT CAMP
5-STEP STRATEGY FOR
INNER AND OUTER STRENGTH

DEVAN KLINE + MORGAN KLINE

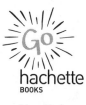

hachette
BOOKS

New York

Hachette Go, an imprint of Hachette Books

Hachette Book Group

1290 Avenue of the Americas

New York, NY 10104

HachetteGo.com

Facebook.com/HachetteGo

Instagram.com/HachetteGo

First Edition: June 2024

Published by Hachette Go, an imprint of Hachette Book Group, Inc. The Hachette Go name and logo is a trademark of the Hachette Book Group.

The Hachette Speakers Bureau provides a wide range of authors for speaking events. To find out more, go to hachettespeakersbureau.com or email HachetteSpeakers@hbgusa.com.

Hachette Go books may be purchased in bulk for business, educational, or promotional use. For information, please contact your local bookseller or Hachette Book Group Special Markets Department at special.markets@hbgusa.com.

The publisher is not responsible for websites (or their content) that are not owned by the publisher.

Print book interior designed by Amy Quinn.

Library of Congress Cataloging-in-Publication Data

Names: Kline, Devan, author. | Kline, Morgan, author.
Title: Burn : the Burn boot camp 5-step strategy for inner and outer
  strength / Devan Kline + Morgan Kline.
Description: First edition. | New York : Hachette Go Books, 2024. |
  Includes bibliographical references and index.
Identifiers: LCCN 2024004157 | ISBN 9780306833694 (hardcover) | ISBN
  9780306833717 (epub)
Subjects: LCSH: Self-actualization (Psychology) | Self-care, Health.
Classification: LCC BF637.S4 K5553 2024 | DDC 158.1—dc23/eng/20240229
LC record available at https://lccn.loc.gov/2024004157

ISBNs: 9780306833694 (hardcover), 9780306833717 (ebook)

Printed in the United States of America

LSC-C

Printing 1, 2024

We dedicate this book to our children, Cameron, Ryan, and Maxwell.
You give us the fire we need to light up the world.
Love you always and forever.

CONTENTS

INTRODUCTION

WE KNOW YOU. YOU'VE COME THROUGH THE DOORS OF ONE OF OUR gyms, Burn Boot Camp, watched us on YouTube, or followed us on social media. You've shared your ups and downs with us at events. You've tried countless diets, exercise, and self-help books, yet you're still not happy with what's happening to your body and your health, or how your life has played out so far. Utterly frustrated, you're someone who has gone through life repeatedly chasing the same goals, or breaking promises to yourself, but never achieving any lasting success. And instead of helping, the health and fitness industry often makes things even worse with unrealistic ideologies, unsustainable plans, and unachievable goals.

You aren't failing to become fit. Fitness is failing you.

What you need are strategies for creating positive, permanent change in your life, and we're here to guide you in that transformation. It will not be about only eating or exercising right. It will be about thinking differently and understanding that your personal health and fitness is your responsibility. This change in your thinking gives you great power and puts you in control of your life, setting in motion one of the most powerful concepts you can learn. *You are entirely up to you.*

Many people don't get this—which is why they have a dismal history of positive change. When life doesn't go their way, they tend to shift the blame and responsibility to external circumstances. Examples: "My whole family is overweight. It's in my genes, so this is just the way I am." Or "It's too cold and rainy to exercise." "I don't have time, with taking care of my kids, family, and everything else."

Statements like these are escape clauses in contracts you can always get out of. Unconsciously allowing yourself to fall into these loopholes swallows up your intentions and motivation, costing you the ownership of your life. **By blaming other people or things, you give away your power.** You then become a victim. You no longer have any control over your life.

We're going to show you how to take back your power, and that means holding yourself accountable for your choices and actions. **When you hold yourself accountable, you set and achieve your goals.** You are more confident. Your life is more organized and less chaotic. **_You_ are in charge. When you're in charge, you make progress, and progress is a key ingredient to happiness.**

Okay, before we go any further, please know that this is not an exercise book, nor is it a diet book. You know most of those books work, yet you are here. Health and fitness are so much more than losing 20 pounds, looking good in a bathing suit, or working out to fit into a dress. We don't even focus on those things. Instead, we want to show you the joy, strength, and health benefits that come from a growth mindset and movement. When you can find joy in movement, and the confidence that comes with mental toughness, you can expect your life to expand in many different ways—with zero pressure to shrink your body. Because the world does not need you to be smaller, quieter, or to be less. The world needs you to show up with everything you have. To build strength and confidence. To set aside guilt and shame and be fully yourself.

What you'll find here is a refreshing approach—one that gives you a less punishing and more sustainable relationship with fitness, whether or not the size or shape of your body changes. You'll never hear us say anything about getting fit so you'll be skinnier and ready for swimsuit season or tiny enough to get into a pair of skinny jeans. But you will hear us talk about the incredible benefits that accrue from fitness, like better sleep, lower stress, increased energy, a reduction in the risk of many diseases, less depression and anxiety, more happiness, and greater success in life.

This book will teach you that your body is not your enemy. Food does not need to be feared. There is a beautiful balanced place where you can replace the time and energy spent struggling with those things with self-confidence, ease, and simplicity. Ask yourself, "What if I loved my body? Finally made peace with it?" What are you giving up by not trying? We promise, you are up to it. We promise you can do this, and you will be amazed.

In this book, we integrate what we call *inner strength* and *outer strength*, combining two things—brain and body, or more accurately, psychology and physiology. Both are deeply, deeply intertwined to create what each of us is truly craving: more energy for a full, satisfying, and happy life.

How exactly are we going to help you achieve that? The journey forward starts with something that probably no one has ever told you to do: move your body daily in challenging, demanding ways. Intentional physical activity is the first step toward taking your life from lukewarm to on-fire living. Where you find your edge is where you'll find *yourself*. Will it be difficult at times? Yes. Will it require courage? Without a doubt. But it's time to let your faith be greater than your fear. It's time to take what's meant for you. It's time to move forward. Motion creates emotion. When you move your body, your brain automatically responds by improving your mental and emotional health in just a single workout.

When you show up and work hard, you'll develop greater confidence. You'll have far less loneliness, depression, and anxiety. You'll feel in control again. You'll have a strong, unchangeable sense of direction. You'll win even when life has dealt you the worst of challenges. You'll feel connected to people. You'll achieve any goal you set for yourself, whether health related, nutritional, financial, relational, or professional. You'll build the life you want from the inside out with one simple, daily action—moving your body.

Unfortunately, many people don't move enough to enjoy those benefits. Statistics say so: more than three-fourths of Americans don't currently hit the CDC's recommended minimum for regular exercise—around 150 minutes a week.

This is a great tragedy of our society because inactivity is self-destructive. On average, people who are physically inactive suffer three or more days of poor mental health each month, including symptoms of stress, depression, anxiety, and other emotional problems. In other words, not moving makes you feel like crap. Stay inactive long enough and that crappy feeling becomes a crappy personality—one you can't even recognize as your own.

This book is full of stories of people who have found themselves in a difficult battle. Battles that felt wholly unwinnable. Ones that took them down to the studs. You'll read about how building inner strength and outer strength saved their lives.

But that might not be you.

Your story might be the one we're most familiar with. Feeling like you're on the hamster wheel of the enormous pressure to get things done and putting yourself dead last. Being the engine that runs everything. Children, career, marriage, friends and family, the house and pets, and playdates and appointments. And even though the engine runs without fail and often on terrible food and not enough water, you still feel an overwhelming sense of guilt for the things you're not. You desperately want to love your life and teach your children that parenthood isn't about misery or martyrdom. You're tired of feeling alone, isolated, putting your goals on the shelf for another year to collect dust. You were active and strong at one point, maybe even an athlete, and you want to feel that confidence again. You want to feel powerful, in control, and fully alive, but you need to figure out where to start.

When people come to us and say something like "I'm stuck" or "I can't move" or "My life is terrible," we fully understand. And yes, it's stuck and terrible today, but it does not have to be that way tomorrow. It's your decision if you want to move and start changing your life. We always say: "You're one decision away from being fulfilled." The one decision we recommend you make to transform *everything* is: work out! **Moving your body is the first step to changing your life.**

So, what's the deal? Why is it that physical activity has such a profound impact on your mental health?

When your body moves, your mind responds. Your feelings, thoughts, motivation, and behavior (inner strength) improve, big-time! Your mind goes where your body leads, not "mind over body," as most fitness books tell you.

What we call "training," or physically demanding activity, is the activation button for many biological effects. One, it releases a cocktail of different brain chemicals that bring about a sense of well-being, happiness, and joy. It also gives you a sense of accomplishment, mastery, and confidence, and creates an overwhelming feeling of aliveness for your spirit.

One of the biggest misconceptions today is that you can simply choose to be happy or successful even in difficult circumstances by "putting your mind to it." As we'll show, the truth is just the opposite. You change by "putting your body to it," first and foremost. Or, as we like to say: outer strength leads to inner strength.

Let's pause here for a second and introduce ourselves. We're the founders, visionaries, and CEOs of Burn Boot Camp, one of the fastest-growing health franchises in the world, with hundreds of gyms all over the United States and beyond. At Burn Boot Camp, we choose not to use mirrors, scales, and monitors traditionally used at gyms because we want our members to concentrate solely on pushing their limits and discovering their inner strength. It's about personal growth and self-belief, not comparison or competition with others. We sincerely believe that these are the things that can derail your fitness journey. That mirror or leaderboard reflects only where you are on that specific day and has nothing to do with where you're headed. Comparison adds a component of competition, and competing with others separates us when what we really need is a community to succeed. Life is a team sport, and we show up to compete with who we were yesterday, rather than the person next to us.

We've created spaces where people can come in, feel welcome, and be inspired by belonging to a community that loves and supports them unconditionally. No one has to set aesthetic goals like getting a bikini bod or shedding a certain number of pounds. They come to know that this is a place where they can have fun and keep progressing toward greater strength, conditioning, mobility, and confidence. Most every fitness program in history has focused on what you need to lose; we focus on everything you can gain.

We're interested in creating lasting change in you. To do that, you must bring three foundational beliefs to the table:

1. I can do this.
2. I must do this.
3. I will do this.

These mantras empower you and kick-start your momentum. When you believe "I can, I must, I will," you're set up to see extraordinary progress with our program because what you believe, you become.

Also, we do a lot more than just teach you how to work out. We teach you how to enjoy eating the right foods—no more going into some crazy, unhealthy state of artificial deprivation. We give you a unique goal-setting system. We teach you how to build community and bond with others. We teach you how to think differently so you can have the life you want. We teach you to put yourself first and train your body hard, which is the ultimate form of self-love and the least selfish thing any of us can do.

In short, we teach you how to do ordinary things that have an extraordinary impact.

Since founding Burn Boot Camp in 2015, from a humbling workout space in a parking lot, we've had the opportunity to affect more than two million people. Their stories are about breakthroughs: coming back from the brink of suicide, recovering from abusive relationships, overcoming alcoholism and other addictions, getting out of financial debt, defying life-destroying diagnoses, and crawling out of many other hit-rock-bottom catastrophes. All they did was decide to believe in themselves and keep moving forward with our program, and they emerged, transformed.

We know all about this because we grew up in worlds with trauma, sadness, and other pretty messy stuff. This is Devan's story:

I grew up in one of the most toxic, abusive environments you can imagine. Being on welfare and living in poverty were the least of my worries—it was hell on earth. My parents beat each other to a pulp on a regular basis. The police were a constant presence on our doorstep at our home at 84 Pleasant Avenue, which turned out to be anything but pleasant. I've watched alcohol and drugs being used in my home nightly. I once found a woman who overdosed in my house and passed away. I've seen a finger get chopped off in a fight, an entire calf muscle ripped off the bone, people get pushed off second stories, heads shoved through glass garage doors, and more. My dad fathered kids by multiple women, all of whom he was physically violent toward. He ended up in jail and prison, not once but multiple times. My mom stole a car I worked hard to buy for myself. She eventually abandoned us and isn't coming back. Over fifty domestic violence charges were filed against my parents before I turned eighteen, from child abuse to assault and battery. These are just the headlines of my childhood—"hell on earth" might be an understatement.

Mine is not a rare story, but it has a rare ending. That's because children exposed to violence are far more likely to abuse drugs and alcohol; suffer from depression, anxiety, and post-traumatic disorders; fail or have difficulty in school; and engage in criminal behavior.

With this kind of past, statistically, I'm not supposed to be here or even make it in life. No male role models, no mentors, no resources—just God and me. I always felt like I was at the starting line of the Boston Marathon in a 100-foot ditch with no ladder.

But you know what? I wouldn't change the way I was raised for anything. My adversity is my advantage. Climbing out of that 100-foot ditch made me the man I am. I decided to turn my struggles into strategies and break the chain of poverty, welfare, and abuse. I was the first one in my family to go to college and graduate. I'm thankful I've experienced pain and was able to use it to create progress.

Thankfully, too, I was also an athlete—in fact, at one time, a pitcher for the San Francisco Giants until a forearm injury and a poor mindset derailed my career. Afterward, I became a personal trainer. Fitness and athletics were all I knew. They freed me from despair, taught me discipline, and transformed my life. If it wasn't for baseball, there's a good chance I wouldn't be here today.

Getting cut from the Giants was a devastating setback, though. It wasn't just the arm injury. I wasn't producing the stats required by the team and my mindset was negative. Plus, even though I was only twenty-three, they wanted to replace me with much younger, even more talented recruits. Something I had worked on my entire life vanished in one moment, and the worst part was that I didn't even see it coming. Feeling defeated, I didn't have a clue about what to do with myself. I was convinced that I was a monumental failure.

Morgan and I met when we were twelve years old. She was my rock (and still is) through the tough times growing up. When my dream ended that day, my first emotion was anger—the next, fear. I was scared that I'd end up like my parents. Naturally, I called Morgan for advice. She said, "Look where you've come from, look at what you've accomplished, and use this to propel yourself. You aren't your parents—keep moving forward." Those words changed my life, and I would do just that—keep moving.

What was my next move? Recalling my time spent living with host families and helping them become healthy and happy during my college and professional baseball years, I spun my love for training into a program inspired by all my experiences. I became an expert at helping people build their inner and outer strength to become something great. That message remains at the heart and soul of Burn Boot Camp.

We were just two kids who grew up in Battle Creek, Michigan, under very different circumstances, but ended up having the same passion. While I was destined to a life of poverty, Morgan was supposed to climb the corporate ladder, be successful, and follow in her family's footsteps. This is Morgan:

I came from a tight-knit and loving family, made tragically smaller when my father died when I was only five. Unlike Devan, I was extremely close to my family and grew up with unconditional love and support. But losing my dad was devastating. My world instantly became scarier and more uncertain, so I made every attempt to control the uncontrollable. I self-isolated out of grief because I felt so different from my friends. I focused on academic success and avoiding unpredictable emotions. I grew up way too fast, feeling an enormous sense of responsibility and obligation to be a success while silencing my own needs.

When we first started Burn Boot Camp, I was a rising star at Kellogg, working my heart out selling sugary cereals and toaster muffins. But pushing processed food felt hollow and unfulfilling, and the harder I worked, the more unrewarding it became. Having been an athlete in high school, I loved being active. I loved the blood, sweat, and tears that went into being a champion. The early mornings, the conditioning drills, and the celebration of the big wins. Being an athlete even helped me begin to cope with the heartbreak of loss. I loved pushing myself to see what my body could do. This passion ultimately made me realize I wanted to pursue a career in fitness.

My first step was into the world of competitive bodybuilding. I got caught up in it, willing to do anything to achieve the same tight, ripped look of female bodybuilders—hard-core fasting, eating boiled chicken breasts when I wasn't starving myself, taking appetite suppressant pills, doing two hours of conditioning and one hour of strength training a day. All of this made me feel miserable, mentally and physically. The worst part was that I began hating my body. I didn't feel worthy, good enough, strong enough, or sexy enough. The whole bodybuilding thing dragged me down until, one day, I broke down. I decided to stop and be my authentic self—no more trying to live up to unattainable media-driven ideals of fitness.

That's when I found true fulfillment—after becoming a personal trainer and inspiring others to change their lives through fitness. I quit my job and committed myself to Burn Boot Camp full-time. Since then, I've personally trained at more than ten thousand camps and am committed to helping people love and accept themselves unconditionally.

In addition to our stories—and other personal stories that will blow you away—we base our plan on powerful, scientifically validated assertions that make this book radically different from others you've read.

Many researchers have looked at the link between health behaviors like exercise and happiness, and they've concluded that regular physical activity is positively associated with greater well-being. For example:

- When you move, your body releases positive chemicals and hormones that relieve stress and make you feel good. You change your brain chemistry and the actions you take.
- When you move, you shake off the mindset of anxiety and negativity, and feel more ready to achieve your life goals.
- When you move, you have a reliable anchor point in your life that makes you feel more in control.
- When you move, you can regenerate brain cells and brain tissue and stave off mental decline caused by age-related brain shrinkage.
- When you move, you meet people and form bonds, especially if you join a gym, attend an exercise class, or walk in a neighborhood park.

Before you start reading, know this: To achieve this level of success is a battle. You either get in the ring, or you watch from the sidelines. If your goal is to be a champion, it's going to be a knock-down, drag-out battle. So, you have to ask yourself: "Is this really a battle I want?" If yes, do you want it badly enough? Are you willing to do whatever it takes? You've got a chance and a choice. It's up to you.

We know you're frustrated with all those exhausting start, stop, start-all-over efforts of the past. You just haven't found the right strategy yet. If you want to live a transformed life—permanently—one filled with the magic you're missing, have the courage to try new things. Life is amazing when you see, live, and embrace new possibilities.

If you're on board with us now, and we hope you are, here's a preview of coming attractions—our program in a nutshell, a proprietary five-point strategic plan:

Burn. Start here. Move and keep moving forward. Don't become sedentary. You *need* to move—it makes an extraordinary difference in your life. It's the best way to remind yourself that *you can do hard things* even when your life is not looking so wonderful right now. Moving your body causes powerful shifts in the way you carry yourself through life. You'll fall in love with fun and rewarding workouts so that they become a source of joy, happiness, social connection, and emotional strength.

To get these benefits, we've created a series of unique workouts you've probably never tried before or even heard of. We want you to go all in with these so that you're left feeling confident and empowered.

Your body will get fitter, your world will get brighter, and your life will get better—beginning with challenging, sweaty, and demanding workouts.

Believe. This is where inner strength is really hammered home. With this strategy, we equip you with psychological tools for sustaining lasting change: how to break negative patterns, identify internal struggles holding you back, adjust your thinking, put yourself first, and create momentum. This strategy keeps you focused and helps develop the inner strength you need for a lifetime of success. We'll show you how your thoughts express themselves as words; your words drive your actions; your actions eventually turn into habits; your habits mold your character; your character shapes your destiny; your destiny becomes your legacy.

Nourish. Feed yourself like you're someone you love. We'll help you find foods that cultivate strength, stamina, and self-confidence without the all-too-familiar feeling of deprivation and restriction. You'll learn how to change your mindset around food—that it's fuel for nourishing your body—a mindset that makes following a healthy nutrition plan completely sustainable. You'll also discover how to take charge of your

nutrition with only five actions, which we call "small wins," that are
life-altering in their simplicity. We believe in "simple." Most plans are too
complicated, and complexity quickly becomes the enemy of execution.

You'll apply our Burn 10-Minute Meal, which can be customized for
anyone. It helps you select the right foods and plan nutritious meals. And
we provide fifty Burn-approved ten-minute recipes. You'll come to enjoy
the wonderful and surprising feeling of being physically active *and* nour-
ishing yourself well.

Achieve. Having goals is critical, but success comes from taking the
focus off the finish line and placing it on the dedication, commitment,
and hard work it takes to cross it. In this book, we take you through a
system that teaches you how to set goals (finding your "why") and how
to create actionable steps to realize them. Those steps are based on our
unique reverse-engineering, goal-setting model that helps you figure out
what to stop, what to start, and what to shoot for in the eight key areas
of your life: your body, mind, emotions, spirit, relationships, time, work,
and money.

Achieving your goals is never a matter of ability. It's always a matter of
inspiration. And the source of that inspiration almost always boils down
to the love you have for the people in your life—and how you keep mov-
ing forward for them.

Connect. You were never meant to do this alone. Your family, friends,
and loved ones are integral to your success. You'll learn how important it
is to allow the people who love you to encourage and support you when
things get hard. Surrounding yourself with people who believe in you and
your goals, who maybe even have the same goals themselves, can be a
huge source of motivation when yours wanes.

But it's more than just an outward connection. You'll begin to connect
to your feelings and needs, your most honest and sincere "why." You'll start
to imagine living a life you love and becoming the person you want to be.

In Part 1, you'll learn about the strategies and what it takes to integrate
them in your lifestyle. In Part 2, we show you how to start living them.
With these five strategies as the foundation, we're excited to share with

you our simple, practical plan, motivated by just the right amount of our signature tough love.

Put these five strategies into play, and you'll transform the person you are now into the person you have the power to become—the person you were always meant to be! Sure, it's hard, but you're worth it.

Rest assured that you're not the guinea pig. At Burn Boot Camp, we've created a massive community who share this outlook on life. This isn't our business. This is something much bigger.

Burn Boot Camp is our lifelong, up-at-dawn, unshakable pursuit to champion men and women and their families. To help those with limiting beliefs understand how truly limitless they are. To convince you that your life is largely in your control, and your past does not define your future. These chapters will prove that becoming powerful in your body can make you powerful in your life. And don't worry if this is your second, third, or even fiftieth attempt to break old patterns. If you failed, you tried, and if you tried, you believed. And belief in yourself is your superpower.

Remember this: You might *seem* stuck, but you're not *really* stuck. We know that, with enough purpose and intention, you can rise above anything. You can completely re-create yourself. You have choices. You can think empowering thoughts. You can reach for lofty goals and get them. You can create healthy habits. No obstacle can crush you. All that matters is that you keep moving forward and show up for yourself and your family every day.

PART 1

INNER AND OUTER TRANSFORMATION

CHAPTER 1

STRATEGY #1: BURN

Lots of people are sedentary—and paying the price with their physical and mental health. Karen was one of them until she developed the consistent, positive habit of working out. She soon discovered that her workouts were doing a lot more for her than just helping her get fit physically.

Karen used to feel a tingle of panic at the thought of exercising. It was intimidating, and she felt too old and too out of shape to consider it. But her daughter Taylor kept pressing and encouraging her to at least try a workout at one of our camps.

"I was embarrassed because I had let myself go, but I had heard good things about it," she said. "So, even though I was terrified, I agreed to give it a go."

In July 2019, Karen walked through the doors of our facility in Monona, Wisconsin. "I peered into the exercise room. They looked like they were having fun."

She joined in. And the most thrilling thing happened. She surprised herself. She was keeping up with the other members in camp, and even though it was one of the hardest things she's ever done, it was *fun*. She fed off the energy in the room and all the high-fives. Her trainer was with her the whole way, reminding her that she could, even when she was sure she *absolutely* could not. "Stay focused," she told herself. "You've got this."

And she did have it. Muscles that had been dormant finally sparked to life, and she felt alive again. "It was great exercise, and I felt like I was not completely terrible at it."

Karen loved the atmosphere, the people, and the ability to modify exercises. She signed a one-year membership and committed herself to five to six workouts a week.

"The first month, I literally cried during every workout, as well as on my car ride home or to work. I was so upset with my body and how out of shape I was. But I knew those tears were from frustration for having given up on myself so many times before. Quitting when it got hard. I wasn't going to let it happen again. I refused to betray myself again."

Encouragement came from everywhere—her trainer, her daughter, the manager, and from all the people in camp.

"One of my first goals was to do a power roll—an exercise in which you lie on your back, roll up until you land on your feet, then jump in the air. Very tough! But with the help of a 20-pound medicine ball for counterbalance, it happened early on in my journey. This gave me the confidence to master other moves."

Over three years, however, Karen faced seemingly insurmountable challenges: plantar fasciitis, sciatica, and a worn-out knee, not to mention the COVID-19 lockdown. In March 2022, she had a total knee replacement, requiring a four-month suspension.

Many people would have given up, but Karen got back in the game, with her trainer guiding her through modifications and pushing her to do more. She felt powerful, knowing what her body could do.

"I've struggled with my weight for 30 years. I've lost more than 50 pounds through exercise, eating reduced meal portions, eliminating sugar, and drinking lots of water," she said. "Not to spout a cliché, but if I can do it, anyone can. It has been baby steps along the way with occasional setbacks, but slow and steady has been working for me. I have a ways to go, and the journey has had its challenges. Still, I feel so much healthier, both physically and mentally, with a much better outlook on my future."

If you had to take only one step toward transforming your life, would you be willing? The Burn strategy is all about doing just that—performing challenging workouts that demand more of you each time you do them. As Karen discovered, change how you move, and you'll change how you feel. You'll begin to appreciate your body for more than just how it looks but as a force of astounding power. You'll be happier, more joyful, and more empowered—someone on top of the world.

Feeling like this will place you in the minority, however! In 2020, for example, an estimated 66 percent of US adults aged eighteen or older underwent treatment for major depression, according to the National Institute of Mental Health. This number is tragic and shockingly high.

Depression isn't just a mental health problem. It wallops the body, causing chronic aches and pain, inflammation, heart disease, insomnia, sexual problems, digestive issues, and weight gain or loss, among others. Depression can eat away at your quality of life and, at worst, send you spiraling down to a mental rock bottom.

Physical movement is intertwined with happiness, positive habits, self-worth, mental outlook, achievement, and social connection. Also, key elements of your character, such as work ethic, discipline, consistency, fortitude, bravery, and so many more, are developed with regular workouts.

We can cite a mountain of studies proving that exercise is the most important tool to blunt everyday stress, anxiety, depression, and other mental pain. Not just to take the edge off, but to completely transform your mental health for the better. But this recent study pretty much says it all.

The study, reported in the *British Journal of Sports Medicine*, covered ninety-seven different analyses over 1,039 trials involving 128,119 participants, making it the most comprehensive review to date. The overall conclusion was that physical activity significantly improves symptoms of depression, anxiety, and distress. Even more impressive was that physical activity is 1.5 times more effective than counseling or taking antidepressants. Two more incredible findings: the benefits of exercise kick in pretty fast—within weeks—and higher-intensity workouts (as we recommend) improved symptoms.

The evidence that exercise changes how you feel is just too overwhelming to ignore. Even the American Psychiatric Association recommends it as a treatment for depression—alone or when used as a multiplier. It enhances the effectiveness of existing therapies, including medications or counseling, by helping people regain happiness and joy.

We agree that challenging workouts are the most underutilized form of antidepressant on the planet; they're the antidote for overcoming many mental obstacles. We should know! Both of us experienced trauma at young ages, and we unpacked it in our own lives through sports and workouts. Exercise is no longer something we should do. It's something we must do! Nor is it nice to have a gym membership or a home gym. It's a need to have.

Great health is a universal human need. You want to feel secure knowing that your body will serve you for years to come. Optimized living is only achieved through moving.

But exactly why is exercise so powerful at improving your outer and inner strength? The Burn strategy offers several surprising insights.

THE BURN STRATEGY HELPS BOOST YOUR MOOD.

The mood boost—usually nicknamed the "runner's high"—that we get from working out is well known. But it's not exclusive to running, nor is it triggered only by the release of feel-good endorphins, as scientists used to think. This incredible mood boost is linked to another set of brain chemicals called *endocannabinoids*.

Endocannabinoids operate like your body's own THC, the most psychoactive substance found in the cannabis plant. Like a key fits into a lock, endocannabinoids latch on to receptors rimmed on cells throughout the body, especially in the brain. After gaining entry into the cells, they reduce anxiety, make you feel calm, and bring about a sense of well-being. They also interact with the brain chemical dopamine, from which you experience pleasure.

One of the healthiest ways to naturally heighten the release of endo-cannabinoids is to move your body and put effort into it. The harder you work out, the greater the release of endocannabinoids and the greater your mood boost. So, to feel really good, you have to go all in!

THE BURN STRATEGY HELPS YOU BREAK BAD HABITS.

We mention habits a lot throughout this book. Brushing your teeth twice a day, going to bed at a specific time, and snacking on certain foods are all habits that you may have developed over time. Habits can be helpful or harmful, depending on the types of habits you have. But what exactly is a habit?

Habits are routines and behaviors that you perform regularly, sometimes without even thinking about them. Some are formed when you deliberately cultivate them; others can develop without your having any intention at all to acquire them. Once habits form, they get locked in the neural pathways of your brain and are often difficult to undo.

Knowing you need to "break" a bad habit is scary because it feels like such a challenge. How do you even begin?

Let's say you're caught up in some of the unhealthiest, most harmful habits, such as bingeing on junk food, drinking to the point of alcoholism, smoking, or taking dangerous drugs. Sure, there are methods and various therapies to help you kick them. But we've got good news for you. Great news. We've witnessed that when demanding workouts are done regularly, they can help even in these critical cases. Before we tell you why, let us introduce you to Hope, from Jupiter, Florida, who broke her addiction to drugs with "sweat therapy." In her words:

When I started attending a Burn Boot Camp in my town, I was battling a twenty-year addiction to smoking cigarettes and taking Adderall, a powerful prescription stimulant. Getting hooked on both was a gradual slide into "uppers," eventually controlling my life. When I first started, I thought I was more productive, confident, and intelligent. But I soon realized I had no power over my need for them and knew the side effects were terrible. Not just terrible, they were killing me. Sitting at a stoplight one day, driving to get yet another pack of cigarettes, I silently prayed that God would show me a way to stop. I looked to my left, and there was this beautiful blue sign, and somehow, I knew instantly he had led me to this place with these people.

Shortly after I started, I had already begun to give up my addictions. I did not want to fall off the wagon and get addicted again, so I was also fully committed to Burn. I can honestly say I have experienced a transformation like no other—mentally, spiritually, and physically. At first, I committed to attending at least four days a week. Now, I'm regularly at camp six days a week without a second thought. The dopamine hit I was getting from the nicotine and Adderall had been replaced with dopamine from exercise. What an incredible gift. I got my life back.

I built a body that I barely recognize but am so very proud of. The people—the trainers and fellow members—are what make this place special. It is possible to become the best version of yourself if you give yourself a second chance, especially if you have any type of addiction. My best advice is to trust the process! I found in my workouts a bright ray of hope. They are life-changing in a huge way. Ironically, ever since I walked into camp and immersed myself in the workouts, I've watched myself rise like a phoenix from the ashes.

There are scientifically validated reasons why working out helps people overcome their addictions and stay off dangerous substances. For one thing, pleasurable activities light up the reward center in your brain. Those sources of pleasure tend to be bad things like drinking alcohol, doing drugs, eating sugary foods, or smoking cigarettes. Stuff that feels good when you're doing it tends to be something you want to repeat again and again, right?

Unfortunately, when you get that "high" from those stimulants, your brain churns out dopamine—the "reward chemical." So, even though you know you're doing something "unhealthy," it's tough to kick because it feels pleasurable in the moment, and your body begins to crave that feeling.

But here's the positive: remember that exercise, too, stimulates pleasurable brain chemicals, such as serotonin, dopamine, and many others, so pretty soon, your brain gets hooked on working out. Exercise becomes a "positive addiction."

Exercising also dulls withdrawal symptoms. You may struggle to kick bad addictive habits because of the physical and emotional distress that hits when the habit is eliminated. Well, more great news. Working out dulls withdrawal symptoms, such as irritability, stress, depression, and restlessness.

In a fascinating experiment reported in the journal *Addiction*, investigators recruited forty sedentary smokers who had smoked at least ten or more cigarettes daily for at least three years. The goal of the study was to find out whether exercise could ease withdrawal symptoms in smokers after they temporarily stopped smoking.

The smokers were randomly put into one of two groups. One group performed ten minutes of moderate-intensity exercise on a stationary bicycle. The other group did not exercise but followed a distraction task (concentrating on something besides smoking) for ten minutes. Both groups abstained from smoking before participating in the experiment. After completing their exercise or task, the smokers rated their withdrawal symptoms and the urge to smoke using certain scales.

At the end of the experimental period, the exercise group had very few withdrawal symptoms. But the other group, which completed the distraction task, still went through withdrawal symptoms. The researchers concluded: "A brief bout of moderate-intensity exercise can lead to a rapid reduction in desire to smoke and withdrawal discomfort. . . . These findings support recommendations that smokers use exercise as a means of helping cope with the difficulties encountered when they try to stop."

If you're dealing with addiction and trying to beat it, working out can help you, and it works as quickly as a single bout of exercise.

THE BURN STRATEGY PROMOTES A LIFE THAT IS PLEASURABLE AND JOYFUL.

When you do something pleasurable, your brain cells release dopamine, a neurotransmitter. Once released, it travels across a gap between nerve cells (neurons) termed a synapse, binds to receptors on nerve cells, and transmits a signal to those cells, all of which culminates in that "Oh, I feel so good" sensation.

Pleasurable things can be good or bad. Bad: any type of substance abuse or behavioral stuff like gambling, pornography, or constantly cruising the internet. Good: exercising, getting out in nature, having sex, to name just a few. Regular exercise, in particular, does two cool things: it keeps dopamine circulating at higher levels and creates more dopamine receptors in cells. With all that happening inside your body, you'll feel more joyful most of the time and definitely less depressed.

On the other hand, bad stuff like abusing alcohol or drugs screws up the dopamine balance in your brain, lowers its levels, and knocks out the number of dopamine receptors on your cells. This chaos is why addicts get depressed, unmotivated, and joyless. Exercise prevents all this!

We've seen this happen so many times in our work. Brian, from our North Suffolk, Virginia, camp, is a great example.

Racing in from long days at the office, Brian would instinctively head to the fridge or the wine rack and open a bottle. Drinking helped the transition from work to evening, and he'd often pour a second glass before dinner. For years, this habit was harmless, or so it seemed.

"I was the funny guy, the life of the party, when I was drinking. It was the way I connected with people. Everyone could always count on me to entertain, be quick with jokes and witty remarks. I felt a sort of responsibility to lighten the mood, which was made much easier with alcohol."

But after about three years, two glasses of wine in the evening became a bottle, a six-pack, or several glasses of bourbon on the rocks. Soon, the alcohol wasn't just at night but also in the late mornings and afternoons.

What Brian didn't realize at the time was that a powerful disease was taking control of his life. Hurt, pain, and disappointment were right on the horizon.

"I'd forget stretches of my day, and there were times when I shouldn't have gotten behind the wheel, but I did. My emotional and physical relationship with my family was absent. I refused to participate in any kind of family activity if it interfered with my drinking. My wife knew something was going on, but I tried to hide the extent of the problem. When she saw how much I was consuming, I would plead for her forgiveness, swearing I'd never touch a drop again, and then start up the next day. I had no control. I was drinking myself to death."

That's the problem with chronic habitual drinking: it's progressive. After a while, alcohol becomes a constant companion, numbing all the bad but all the good too. Until something catastrophic happens and convinces you to boot it out.

That's what happened to Brian. His wife was going to divorce him.

That was enough to get him into treatment for alcohol abuse. He would not let his marriage crumble under the weight of his addiction. He was going to fight like hell for his family *and for himself.* On the recommendation of his therapist, Brian began exercising at one of our locations. Exercise has long been advised if you're trying to quit alcohol and drugs because it diverts your attention away from cravings and eases withdrawal symptoms. But most of all, it rewires the brain's pleasure centers to revive proper dopamine action.

Brian worked tirelessly and met 100 percent of his goals. He stopped drinking, restored his health, repaired his relationships, and regained control of his life. He was so unbelievably grateful for the difference his workouts made in his life he started his own Burn Boot Camp in his community to help others do the same.

As Brian's story shows, the biological response to demanding workouts is unparalleled.

THE BURN STRATEGY IS A CONFIDENCE BUILDER.

Have you ever wondered how you present yourself when you enter a room? Are you slouched over, or are you in a shoulders-back power position? Is your posture commanding or soft and weak? The way you carry yourself displays your self-confidence or lack thereof.

Self-confidence is a belief in your worthiness. That you're good at certain things, have the courage to make tangible improvements in yourself, and achieve success in your life. It also shows up in how you carry yourself.

Think of self-confidence as the electricity in your home. You may not know every detail about how it works, but it's frustrating when it's off. Just as when your power goes out, a lack of self-confidence has a huge adverse impact on inner and outer strength.

Fortunately, you can do a lot to shore it up. One massive piece of the confidence puzzle is exercise. Research has shown that people who are more active are more self-confident.

How so?

Here's an example: You go from being barely able to do one push-up in the gym to eventually doing twenty-five one-arm push-ups with ease. That's an empowering feeling because you are literally stronger and more skilled now. While exercise makes you more capable of doing physical things, that sense of physical strength crosses over into all areas of your life. This is where the gains in outer strength translate to greater confidence in other areas of your life. You started something that felt challenging, maybe even impossible, and yet you believed in yourself and achieved it. You proved to yourself through exercise that you can set tough goals, working toward them and achieving them. You'll even feel braver and more courageous, emboldened to make a career change, tell someone you love them, or stand up for yourself.

The ease of using your workouts as a tool to build confidence is really the magic. Everyone has great days and not-so-great days. The easiest thing to do is show up and move your body, regardless of how you're feeling. This is what makes you unstoppable. This is what helps you get where you want to go. This is what makes you succeed in whatever you set out to do.

Along the way, you'll find that daily worries just don't seem so burdensome. Work stresses are not so intimidating, partly because exercise downregulates levels of stress hormones in your body, such as adrenaline and cortisol. Relationship problems are not so problematic. One day, you'll wake up and realize that you're living the life you always wanted.

Confidence is your superpower. Once you believe in yourself, accept yourself unconditionally, and stop judging yourself, that's when your life begins to change. The most exciting element of confidence is that it's an ability, a skill you can acquire. Demanding workouts are the best tool to develop your confidence and kick-start your momentum.

THE BURN STRATEGY SUPPORTS BRAIN HEALTH.

To build a healthy brain, work out!

The brain is like a muscle, but only in the sense that it typically shrinks with age—in some areas by as much as 25 percent. This isn't a new, eye-opening breakthrough in science. Years ago, researchers in Scotland assessed the IQ of every Scottish child born in 1936. At age seventy, 691 of those same children completed a survey about their lives and levels of physical activity.

Three years later, researchers analyzed their brain scans at the University of Edinburgh, looking for visible indications of cognitive decline.

The results were shockingly irrefutable. The subjects who exercised regularly over time had less brain shrinkage and fewer structural signs of cognitive decline. This is powerful proof of how physical activity reduces risk factors, keeps your mind active, and keeps you at the top of your game as you get older.

Regular exercise also reduces chronic inflammation (which can attack the brain). It releases chemicals that help improve the health of brain cells, and supports the growth of new blood vessels that feed the brain with oxygen and nutrients.

Working out nourishes the hippocampi, a pair of seahorse-shaped structures within the brain. (*Hippocampus* is the Greek word for "seahorse.") They're responsible for memory formation. Long-term memories are routed through them prior to being stored in the brain. If the hippocampi shrink or lose volume, memory problems, cognitive decline, and even Alzheimer's disease can set in.

One of the best ways to nourish these structures and protect your brain is to get moving. Working out shields the hippocampi from chronic stress (which will shrink them) and increases their volume. When it comes to memory and learning, you want more hippocampi cells.

Regular physical activity also boosts the production of brain-derived neurotrophic factor (BDNF). This specialized protein is essential for healthy brain cells, learning, and memory. It may also shield your brain from age-related mental decline. In fact, just six minutes of strenuous exercise can quintuple the production of BDNF!

This protein also supports neuroplasticity (the ability of the brain to continue growing and be molded in response to life experiences), and is associated with easing depression and anxiety.

With a healthy brain, boosted by regular workouts, you'll get mental clarity. That's something we believe is necessary to achieve your goals, stay focused, and define a meaningful purpose in your life. You really don't have your stuff together until you have a healthy body and mind. Notice we say body first and mind second. The term "mind-body connection" is backward because how we move determines how we think.

THE BURN STRATEGY HELPS YOU SLEEP BETTER.

Most of us are awake around sixteen hours a day. If you want to be your best, most vibrant self during that time frame, quality sleep is a must.

Sleep is a physical, mental, and emotional recovery process. Without enough quality sleep, you increase your chances of being depressed, developing high blood pressure, putting on weight, and even risking premature death.

There are lots of strategies you can try to improve lousy sleep patterns. But the best is regular exercise. Exercise gives you more restorative slumber, especially during deep and rapid eye movement (REM). During deep sleep, the brain flushes out toxins that have accumulated during the day, consolidates your memories, and replenishes energy stores (this is important because the brain consumes about 20 percent of your body's energy).

The more active REM sleep starts to dominate as the night goes on. A lot happens during REM sleep. It helps you become a better learner. You have vivid dreams. Your limbs become temporarily paralyzed so that you don't act out your dreams. Your brain processes emotions during REM sleep. Your central nervous system is activated, preparing your body to wake up.

All stages of sleep need to be normal for the brain and body to stay healthy and functioning at peak levels. So, exercise hard and sleep well. It's a great formula for a great life.

THE BURN STRATEGY BUILDS BONDS
AND STRENGTHENS MOTIVATION.

One reason we've seen so many transformations in our camps is that we bring people into an environment where moving their body with other like-minded people is fun. They feel that they're part of a team. Working out with a group of other people is an enormously powerful way to stay motivated, be consistent, improve your performance, find support and accountability, and have fun at the same time.

What you may not realize, though, is that group workouts provide a big mental edge over solo workouts. Exercising with other people releases a hormone called oxytocin, known as the bonding or love hormone. This is exactly what it does. It helps people bond with one another. One study found an uptick in oxytocin levels, measured in people's saliva, after high-intensity martial arts training.

Another reason group exercise is so powerful is that there is a measurable electromagnetic energy field surrounding every human being. Most of this energy is emitted by your heart. In fact, the heart's energy is said to extend nearly 3 feet outside the physical body, according to *Psychology Today*. So, in a group exercise class, we feel one another's positive energy, and from it, we gain joy, strength, and inspiration in community.

So, imagine this: You're in a group exercise setting. Everyone is sweating and pushing their way through a tough workout. Everyone is moving in sync. And everyone is churning out oxytocin and feeling one another's energy like crazy. The overall effect is that everyone in the group feels closer to one another. There is a rush of collective joy, happiness, and connection when you gather together like this—and this collective energy has been documented by scientists who study groups that gather together to incite riots or create peace, as well as exercise together.

Also, it's just more fun to work out with other people! Scientists from the University of Southern California discovered that those who worked out with friends (or a spouse or coworker) reported that they enjoyed the exercise more than those who sweated it out alone.

Our workouts, both in this book and in our camps, are novel and different from most everything out there because they are fun. You never do the same workout twice. You change it up all the time. This builds momentum, breaks through your plateaus, keeps you interested and motivated, develops new muscle faster, and most importantly, builds your inner strength.

OKAY—WHAT'S IT GOING TO TAKE?

How you do one thing is how you do everything. The most practical "one thing" you can do is to perform demanding workouts. Maybe you've wanted to be more active for a long time, but you haven't done anything about it. Well, it's time to stop sitting on the sidelines and get into the game. Here's what it takes.

Be Consistent

Important decisions show up in two places: your calendar and your bank account. You can say, "This is my priority," but you only have to look as far as last year's calendar and your checking account to see what you truly value.

Consistency over everything. It's one of our mottoes! And it's nonnegotiable. That means making your weekly workouts the anchor in your schedule. If fitness is number ten on your list, you'll give it a tenth-place effort. If it's your priority, you'll give it a first-place effort. Working out becomes real only when it's on your schedule and you show up. If your workouts are sporadic, you won't see or feel results. So, schedule them to be consistent.

Changing your language makes you more consistent too. Often we use the statements "I should do that" and "I will do that." They differ by only one word, but that one word makes all the difference in your level of commitment.

When you say you "should" do something, you're really saying *I know I should, but I'm not going to*, making "should" a pretty lame word. When it comes to doing the stuff that matters, "will" has all the punch. When we say we "will" do something, it expresses a commitment. There is no "maybe," no "might," no "I'm thinking about it." The major decision (to do it or not do it) has already been made.

For consistency, it's also critical to do what keeps you in the game: that it's something you enjoy and doesn't feel like a chore. Our workouts do all of that, and more. They're fun, they change things up, they boost your energy and mental strength, and of course, they change your inward experience.

Also, it's important to reframe how you think about working out. Remind yourself of all the great physical, emotional, and mental benefits you get from workouts. Embrace the hard work. Welcome the discipline.

Project how you'll feel after training as opposed to focusing on the training itself. When you do that, you'll be consistent.

Many people stay consistent because they love to prove to themselves they can do it, and they enjoy the hard work involved in tackling these challenges. There's an appeal in pushing yourself hard. Waking up every day with the growth mindset to "do something in the gym I've never done before" will make your progress and happiness inevitable.

If you're like many, you love finding your limit. Yet you never really know where that limit is unless you exceed it. That's something a lot of us search for in life. Finding that point from which we can push past in our workouts helps us to carry on in similar ways in our personal lives.

Make Yourself Number One

We're talking about making yourself a priority. This isn't a luxury either. We'll go as far as to say it's a moral responsibility because your body is such a beautiful blessing.

Think about it. Your heart beats and pumps life through your system without your even realizing it. Your immune system is fighting off cellular invaders you don't even know are attacking. That 3-pound mass of wrinkly material in your skull regulates every single thing you do, from thinking, learning, creating, remembering, and feeling emotions to controlling every blink, breath, and heartbeat. Your body is perfect and brilliant for what it does every single day and not what it looks like in skinny jeans! Yet we live in a culture that undervalues taking care of the body.

As a result, too many people treat their body as if it's broken, when really their body isn't broken at all; their belief in themselves is. You are the most intelligent, resourceful, and beautiful creature known to exist, and best of all, you have a mind. Your mind is equipped with all the tools you need to change. But you can only change you if you believe you're worthy and have a vision of the person you want to become. All the transformation stories you've read so far have one thing in common;

Karen, Hope, and Brian had all lost themselves. But through their commitment to caring for their bodies, there was a ripple effect throughout their whole lives. They finally realized that when we take care of ourselves, we take care of our people. Believe in yourself, believe you are worthy, and you'll act accordingly.

Recognize What You Can Control and Accept What You Can't

Neither of us grew up in ideal situations. We realized that we didn't choose them; we were placed in them. We couldn't control external circumstances, other people, their choices, or their judgment of us. But there were aspects of our lives that we could control: our thoughts, emotions, actions, and the meaning we chose to give to the events in our lives.

As we became passionate about fitness and building our company, we discovered that workouts are one of the few things that we can control in our lives, even when the economy is going to hell, a pandemic hits, or when things are sideways with a job or a relationship.

Human beings desire predictability. But the problem is that life isn't predictable. So much of life is out of your control—the actions of others, the past, the future, events, what happens around you, what others think of you, and so forth. For a lot of what you do in life, someone else has influence. But your workouts? You're in charge!

You're also the boss of your beliefs and behaviors, the goals you set, how you speak to yourself, what you give your energy to, how hard you work, the attitude you bring, and how you respond to challenges and events.

Don't chase what you can't control. This will lead only to frustration. It's also exhausting, not to mention disempowering. For peace of mind, focus only on what you can control, and let the other aspects of life play out without wasting your energy. You don't have the power to dictate everything in your life, but you certainly have the power to choose how you respond to life's circumstances, and to decide whether to stress over them or let them go.

Say Yes to Hard Things

Sure, getting started in a workout program or upping your effort in a current workout can be hard. But at Burn Boot Camp, one of our affirmations is "Say yes to hard things." And that includes our workouts.

As challenging as our workouts are, you can do them, even if you start small, with modifications, and progress from there. If it doesn't challenge you, it won't change you, and that goes for everything in life.

Think about the last time you were scheduled for a workout. What was zooming through your mind? We bet you were murmuring some derivative of "No, no, no, this is going to be hard. I don't want to go . . ."

But if you go anyway, you've just said yes. And guess what? You'll finish with a sense of joy, feel-good chemicals pumping through your body, and a rush of accomplishment, and pretty soon you've made a habit of doing positive things that once weren't so comfortable. Saying yes is a lifestyle.

Saying yes to hard things is really about your mental view. Your "hard things" in life are whatever you think they are—like getting up before sunrise to exercise even when you want to sleep in, traveling to a new country, volunteering to take on a project at work that nobody else was willing to do—anything, really, that you've normally avoided doing. All these things make a difference and essentially make you a better, healthier, happier, and more fulfilled person.

Coaches used to tell us: "Practice harder than you play." What they meant was, how you prepare for life's challenges is a reflection of how you handle them. Life favors the prepared, those who are willing to voluntarily do hard things and prepare mentally and physically for them. When you do hard things, *you're strengthened in ways that you then carry into multiple parts of your life, and ultimately situations are easier to handle.*

Life will be hard either way, so choose your hard. It's harder to say no because you risk living a life that has no real meaning for you. "No" is negative. "No" is the beginning of nothing. "No" keeps you stuck. There is no positivity, joy, kindness, or optimism to experience when you say no.

We encourage you to say yes to hard things—all the things that scare you, the things that yank you out of your comfort zone, the things you don't want to do. Say to yourself, "I don't want to be safe. I want a change."

We agree with Richard Branson, who says, "Life is a hell of a lot more fun if you say yes rather than no."

This is how it is for us and how we know it can be for you. It all starts with the decision to make some positive changes, eliminate obstacles, and embrace a new challenge. You're going to love where this takes you.

CHAPTER 2

STRATEGY #2: BELIEVE

As you begin your own transformation, think about the miraculous metamorphosis in nature from caterpillar to butterfly. Before plump little caterpillars turn into winged works of art, they first digest themselves, dissolving into a mush called "the pupal soup." In much the same way, we're at different stages of our own transformations—some of us still unformed, some of us already successfully and beautifully emergent—like Tori.

Not long ago, Tori was a shell of the person she used to be well before she joined our Burlington, Wisconsin, camp. A severe alcoholic, if she was awake, she was drinking. To get out of bed, she was drinking. To work, she was drinking. Yet her family had no idea how bad her addiction was because she still managed to function and was extremely careful to hide her habit.

I tried to maintain my life, my job, home, relationships, etc., but it was so hard. I had to drink before work just to settle myself before the DTs set in, and then worry all day that my coworkers could smell the alcohol on my breath. I'd have more around lunchtime just to make it to 5 p.m., when my time was my own and I could drink until I passed out.

I developed a tolerance so high, I could drink more than any man I know and still be standing. Every day, alcohol was sitting on my shoulder like a demon, reminding me who the boss was. The drink. It was degrading, exhausting, and frightening. I knew I was killing myself, but the thought of that was preferable to living without drinking. I eventually lost my will to live. The drinking had consumed me.

Tori's suicidal thoughts escalated, going from occasional to daily. After a night of severe bingeing, she somehow managed to call her brother, and off they sped to the emergency room.

My blood alcohol concentration was so high that the doctor couldn't believe I was conscious. I was whisked off to a detox clinic, where I spent the next several days in a hospital bed, convulsing, vomiting, and hallucinating. In the days that followed, I met a kid who had barely survived a heroin overdose. Another man cried to me about being too high on crack to attend his son's birthday party. And I realized that I was no different than them. Addiction is addiction, no matter how you slice it.

After detoxing, despite the white-knuckle experience of fresh sobriety, Tori made several positive lifestyle changes. She moved away from the town she lived in, where many of her triggers remained. She started walking every day and changed her diet. She felt good but wanted to feel even better.

One day, Tori's mother asked whether she wanted to attend a ribbon-cutting ceremony at a new Burn Boot Camp location in Herriman.

I said, "Hell, no!" I had never worked out a day in my life. I used every excuse in the book to avoid participating in high school gym class! I had been a music and art nerd my whole life. Well, I did go, but kicking and screaming all the way. It was so foreign to me. What in the actual "f" was I doing there?

It didn't take long for Tori to realize that she wasn't out of place after all. And sure enough, challenging exercise was a miracle for her.

And, although I still can barely do a burpee or wall sits, I am stronger than I ever have been. And not just physically—my journey has been far more mental.

The past year has been a hell of a ride, and my journey is far from over. Hell, it probably never will be. I'm just grateful to have my family, my friends, my puppies, my art and music, and, last but not least, Burn for helping me rise from the ashes. The devil manifests itself in addiction, but at least now I'm a lot stronger to fight back.

Tori woke up almost every day of her life tortured by suicidal thoughts and hooked on alcohol. Her adult life had been an ongoing struggle with addiction, depression, anxiety, and chronic suicidal ideation.

You may not be dealing with an addiction or thoughts of suicide, but you may be troubled by a lot of negativity in your life.

What if you woke up every morning thinking about your worries, your pains, your stresses, people you're mad at, and your problems? How do you think you'll perform that day? Where does your focus go when this happens? Well, guess what? You'd become what you think about most of the time. Thinking about everything that's going wrong invites bad outcomes into your life.

Tori did the opposite. She first got off alcohol. She then got her body moving for the first time ever, and the game began to change. When she did that, she regained control of her emotions. With that, she took control of her attitude. She began to change her beliefs, especially about herself. She changed her focus from "How did I get to such a bad place in my life?" to "How am I going to take control of my life?"

A subtle change in focus from a negative to a positive like that can shift your whole world!

When you look for reasons to succeed, you're going to find them. When you look for reasons to fail, you'll find them too. Where you place your focus determines your direction.

Think of the horses in the Kentucky Derby. In addition to their superhero-like masks, they wear blinders to prevent them from looking to their side. They can only see what's in front of them. Why? Because if they focus on the other horses, they will lose a step.

When you turn your attention to the wrong things, you're going to derail your success. If a horse looks left or right, it may lose its chances to win. If you lose your focus, winning is less of an option.

The Burn strategy we just talked about indirectly shapes your inner strength. But Believe is the strategy that directly develops it. If you're in a bad place right now, the Believe strategy will rescue you. If you're in an awesome place, this strategy will take you to the next level. It is for anyone who desires to reach their maximum potential. We promise you that it will help you install new thinking, new belief systems, and new self-management strategies, truly in the sense of reprogramming your brain.

Ever feel simply on fire? If so, your mind and body are aligned perfectly. Your physical training sets the stage for your mental health to perform well, and you feel congruent. You're disciplined, and you have everything rolling. You're flowing with positive energy and operating life at a productive, high frequency and connected to something greater than yourself.

When your brain and body are congruent like this, magic happens. You can navigate the world and become as happy, successful, and joyful as you desire because your primary state of being is driven by positive emotion.

Unfortunately, the default setting in the human brain is to think in a negative way. Seldom do we think about the things we like and that make us happy—such as being grateful, having purpose, liking ourselves and others.

This default state can be overwhelming unless you do something about it—which is where the Believe strategy comes in. It teaches you to focus on what you want rather than what you don't want. The emotional lens through which you view life controls your state of mind. If you can get clear with your emotions and their power over your perspective, you can change your life.

You want to be successful, don't you? If you want to be successful, for example, be healthier, build an illustrious career, have loving relationships or any desire, focus on these things! Don't let fear, doubt, or negativity mess with it! It's your decision where to place your focus. Every decision you make and every thought that goes through your head moves you closer, or further away, from your destiny.

With this strategy, you'll reprogram your psychology, install new belief systems, and take your life to a whole new level.

THE BELIEVE STRATEGY DEVELOPS YOUR EMOTIONAL INTELLIGENCE.

Emotional intelligence is the ability to express and handle your emotions in a healthy way. Being emotionally intelligent benefits every part of your life, from relationships to your health, and has been shown in studies to increase happiness and longevity.

Emotionally intelligent people share a variety of traits. They:

- Can read other people's emotions
- Are empathetic, able to identify and describe what others are feeling
- Know their personal strengths and limitations
- Are self-confident and self-accepting
- Remain resilient in the face of adversity and make decisions sensitively
- Manage their emotions in a healthy way or in tricky situations
- Have strong relationships

- Accept responsibility for their mistakes (no victim thinking)
- Accept and embrace change

Can you build emotional intelligence? Yes—forget the old ripped abs six-pack and develop a far more important six-pack of emotional intelligence:

Self-awareness. Know yourself and your feelings. Understand what triggers you and how you react to different situations. When you're self-aware, you can better manage your emotional responses.

Emotional regulation. Learn to keep your emotions in check and express them in a healthy way. Recognize when you're living in negative emotional states, and work on ways to control your impulses and reactive behaviors. In a study of centenarians, the ability to express emotions was found to be a common trait, along with a positive attitude toward life, among those living to age one hundred and older.

Empathy. Put yourself in someone else's shoes and try to understand their needs and feelings. Empathy helps us connect with others and maintain strong relationships by listening to what others are needing and feeling.

Conflict resolution. Conflict resolution in emotional intelligence is an empathetic, collaborative resolution of disagreements. It involves active listening, understanding emotions, and finding mutually satisfactory solutions while maintaining positive relationships.

Resilience. When was the last time you went through a loss, a setback, or a major disappointment? How did you handle it? By dwelling on the disappointment? Or did you find a faint flash of positivity amid the darkness—a silver lining of some sort? How fast did you bounce back? In other words, how resilient were you?

Emotionally intelligent people have a bounce-back quality—the ability to adapt to difficult situations and rebound from them, sometimes more strongly than before. Resilient people also tend to be optimists; their positive thinking can undo the effects of a negative experience. Disappointment and pain are sacred lessons. So, stay positive and remember that tough times don't last forever.

Gratitude. Practice gratitude daily by recognizing and appreciating the good things in your life. Gratitude lights a fire in your mind, body, and spirit that not even a dreadful day can put out.

Emotional intelligence is a skill, and as such, you can strengthen it through practice. A big part of this is first identifying the emotions you're having, as well as what is behind them. Once you're in touch with your emotions, you can handle whatever ups and downs come your way. In our view, emotional intelligence is one of the single most important skills you can learn to navigate a purpose-driven, passionate, and meaningful life.

THE BELIEVE STRATEGY TEACHES YOU TO THINK DIFFERENTLY.

Whatever you believe and think about becomes your reality. There is nothing magical about this, and it's been this way since the beginning of consciousness. It is simply the way our brain operates and stems from an amazing tool in your brain called the reticular activating system (RAS).

This small part of your brain is a bundle of neurons located in the brain stem at the base of your skull. Its job is to help you focus on what's important to you. Whatever you think about during the day, positive or negative, you will most definitely find or experience. Put another way, "Seek and you shall find." Sound familiar?

If you think about achieving fitness success, you'll tune in to the right information to make it happen. If you think fitness success isn't important, you'll find perfectly valid reasons to justify why you're not pursuing it. The RAS helps you see what you want to see, and in doing so, influences your actions.

Also, what you believe you deserve is what you will always get. A good example has to do with lottery winners. Ninety percent of people who win the lottery go broke. Let that sink in for a moment. Why? Because they didn't change their thoughts and beliefs about themselves. They never believed they were rich or wealthy. And so, they sabotaged themselves by never altering their inner narrative. Their thoughts and beliefs led them down the path of feeling worthless and eventually going broke.

Your mind is very powerful. When you know exactly what you want, and you think about it constantly and believe you can have it, read about it daily, and talk about it with others, you'll begin to attract what's in alignment with that future. Thinking like this is a much better strategy than just saying you're going to eat less and exercise more. Let your RAS get you there instead. It's your decision where to place your focus, and every decision moves you closer or further away from your destiny. If you're open to thinking differently, you'll get different results.

THE BELIEVE STRATEGY USES THE WORDS OF WINNERS, NOT THE LANGUAGE OF LOSERS.

All of us have an internal voice with unconscious language patterns; sometimes it spills out verbally. Is your dialogue a winning or losing dialogue?

Often referred to as "self-talk," this dialogue ranges from random observations about our environment to criticisms about what we look like, how we're treated, or whether we can accomplish something.

The truth is that our self-talk and day-to-day language have a huge influence on the way we see ourselves, and whether we experience success in life. Our language patterns are proof of whether we are pessimistic or optimistic. It's evidence of our attitude, effort, and strength of belief.

Much of our ongoing internal conversation, however, is negative. The language you use (especially small, seemingly insignificant words) influences and intensifies everything, good or bad, including the actions you take. A few examples:

Using words like *if*, *try*, or *hope* automatically creates doubt and uncertainty. Have you ever said: "I hope I can lose weight"? This is a common expression people use. But by eliminating the single word *hope*, you change the entire meaning of what you said. A word like *hope* gets in the way of reaching any worthwhile goal. Life is black-and-white; either you do it or you don't.

Instead, use the word *when*. *When* presumes that something will be done, whereas *if* leaves it to chance. "When I get my body back . . . when I get that promotion . . . when I do this." A simple switch to the word *when* motivates you to take action.

Watch out for phrases like "I will try" too. If you use this expression, you've already given yourself permission to fail! No matter what happens, you can always claim that you "tried." Want to achieve your goals? Never say "I will try."

Another word trap is using *should* rather than *must*. People say *should* a lot. I *should* get to the office earlier. I *should* eat better. I *should* work out every day, and I *should* do this or that. We *should* ourselves into doing practically nothing!

Trade the word *should* for *must*. If you say you *must* eat healthier or you *must* work out every day, this becomes a definition of our true behavior rather than an imaginary version of how it should be. *Must* is a powerful transformative word that implies there is no other option but to take action toward your goals.

When you have strong inner strength, you habitually practice the words of winners. Talking to yourself and using language in ways that are empowering can transform your life. Here are few language swaps to get you started. Trade:

- "I'm fine" for "It's an amazing day and I'm grateful."
- "I don't know" for "Yes" or "No." Not knowing is passive.
- "I might try to do it" for "I will do it." Trying is a bad strategy!
- "I have to have that" for "I will have that."
- "I've failed so many times in the past" for "I will succeed in the future."
- "I blew it; I'm done" for "No one is perfect. I will learn from my experience."

- "This is horrible" for "This is a beautiful lesson."
- "If it weren't for my situation, I could get fitter" for "No one else can make me fit besides me."
- "I will get back on my plan on Monday" for "I will get back on my plan right now."

Recognize how words—what you say verbally and in your mind—affect your life. We are going to teach you to install "the gap" from the thoughts you think to the words you speak. In this gap is where emotional intelligence lives and you can apply it. Think of "the gap" like hiring a 7-foot bouncer to stand guard at the doorway of your mind and allow only positive, affirming thoughts to enter the party. The most powerful aspect of this is that over time, you can condition yourself to recognize that the language of losers isn't serving you, but you can replace it with the words of winners!

THE BELIEVE STRATEGY ACTIVATES THE MAGIC OF MOMENTUM.

When it comes to creating inner strength, momentum is everything. By definition, it is the strength or force that something has when it's moving forward. As it moves, it grows stronger or faster with the passage of time. Isn't that what you want to make your life work?

The people with momentum who accomplish the most are those who focus on putting physical, mental, emotional, and spiritual strategy into action—quickly, consistently, and aggressively. Focusing on changing yourself from the inside out to become a success in life is destination number one.

Gaining momentum starts with a belief about what's possible for your life. That level of belief determines the actions you take. If you take massive action in all these areas, you'll get massive results. Once you get those results, you boost your belief in yourself. You'll take even more action, yielding even greater results. This is the magic of momentum.

OKAY, WHAT'S IT GOING TO TAKE?

The Believe strategy aligns your physical, mental, emotional, and spiritual mindset to create inner strength. All the scattered pieces of your life come together, and your impetus for getting fit and healthy takes on new meaning. You want to change, you do change, and you change permanently. To begin that journey:

Power Up Your Attitude, Effort, and Beliefs

There are three keys that strengthen your mental muscle: your attitude, effort, and beliefs. All three are completely under your control. That's good news because, as we said, a lot of life is outside our control. We can't control government policies. We can't control what our loved ones think of our career path. We can't control wars or acts of terrorism around the globe. The only thing you can control is yourself. You can control your attitudes, how much effort you put into something, and what you believe in.

What exactly is "attitude"? It's simply the perspective we bring to life every day—a lens through which we interpret our world and our version of reality. Sometimes, that lens is positive; other times, it's negative.

A story that's made the rounds concerns a man who worked for a circus. His job was to clean up after elephants. A coworker watched him in this job and couldn't hold back his perspective. "You have the worst job of anyone I know. You scoop up the elephants' mess every day. It's so demeaning. Why don't you quit?"

The guy working for the circus said, "What? And give up show business?"

It's not what we do so much that matters, it's our attitude toward it. When you're constantly brooding and thinking negatively, your attitude will never change, and soon all that negativity begins to spread around you like wildfire. You'll feel depressed, sad, and unhappy.

You've got to work on changing your daily focus. Instead of focusing on negative events and how bad things are in life, focus on the things you are grateful for. That simple change in your attitude better equips you to deal with any negatives in your life.

Your attitude is driven primarily by positive or negative emotion. It can determine whether you succeed or fail, whether you enjoy life or muddle through it. It greatly influences your body, mind, emotions, spirit, relationships, time, work, and money.

With a positive attitude, you can improve the quality of your life in all eight of these areas. Conversely, if you maintain a negative or skeptical attitude, you will not be able to achieve the life you desire.

Everyone wants to be happy. So, why aren't you happy right now? It's quite simple. The roadblock is a negative or pessimistic attitude.

In his book *Learned Optimism*, well-known psychologist Martin Seligman wrote:

> The defining characteristic of pessimists is that they tend to believe that bad events will last a long time, will undermine everything they do and are their own fault. The optimists, who are confronted with the same hard knocks of this world, think about misfortune in the opposite way. They tend to believe that defeat is just a temporary setback or a challenge, that its causes are just confined to this one case. The optimists believe that defeat is not their fault: Circumstances, bad luck, or other people brought it about. Such people are unfazed by defeat. Confronted by a bad situation, they perceive it as a challenge and try harder.

So, do you see yourself as an optimist or pessimist?

This question—and indeed your answer—is really important to your health and fitness journey. Research has repeatedly shown that optimists are generally healthier than pessimists. For example, optimists have a 50 percent lower risk of heart disease and higher survival rates when dealing with cancer. But pessimism? Some studies have linked it to higher rates of viruses, declining health, and earlier death.

Seligman also found that optimism is the most important predictor of success and happiness. It determines the direction in which your life will go.

As for effort, this is the energy you put in to make something happen. When you put effort into something, impressive results always follow, and they are compounded. Achieving results reinforces your belief in your potential, which leads to even more positive results.

Putting forth effort flows from an optimistic attitude. Sure, a pessimist might be super talented, but if they don't have an optimistic outlook, it's practically impossible to gather up effort.

Devan here: "I describe myself as a radical optimist. I believe in myself and in unlimited potential. I didn't have a lot of talent, but I believed I could play professional baseball. My attitude led to my putting effort in the gym and with my nutrition. I gained 25 pounds of muscle and increased my fastball into the low to mid-90s because of the effort. Everyone around me was more naturally gifted, but I outworked everyone around me all the time."

Here's the moral of the story: when attitude meets effort, you can do anything you put your mind to.

That said, we're all going to run up against negative parts of our society. You can't change this stuff. All you can do is change yourself—your attitude and your effort.

On March 23, 2020, during the pandemic, we were forced to shut down 275 gyms. Our company was worth more than $100 million. That's life-changing value for us. Shutting down forced us to stare in the face of plummeting to $0 in value.

For thirty seconds, we went into a pessimistic default mode. We thought our future was going to vanish. Then we shifted our attitude. We began to believe this was the best thing that could have ever happened to us. We told ourselves: "When times get really bad, this is our opportunity to become *great*."

We broadcast a video to our franchise partners with a single message to bring our belief to them. We asked them to "hold the line." This meant that we would show up for our members, no matter what.

So, we did a bunch of innovative stuff. For one thing, we live-streamed our workouts. Guess what? Fifty thousand people showed up at the first event!

We delivered our nutritional products and activewear on doorsteps. Our franchise partners and trainers used Zoom locally every day.

We felt that we would not only survive but thrive during this time. Our effort reflected this attitude, and results followed. We grew 12.5 percent through the pandemic when all our major competitors' sales plummeted.

Today, our brand value has more than quadrupled—because our attitude and effort led to huge geometric results for the company as well as continued wellness for members in a time they needed us most. Instead of the pandemic crushing us—it created us.

We refused to let a failing economy be our economy, and here's what we learned: Push through adversity; don't let it push you. Never give up. Take a "zero quit" attitude. There is always a way if you get resourceful—even when there are no resources. Get creative—open up your mind.

You can't really conquer a pandemic. You conquer yourself. You overcome the obstacle, your fears, or your self-doubt to move to the next level.

Our success amid adversity also stemmed from our belief system. A belief system drives what you do or don't do. It's a set of principles made up of attitudes, efforts, and beliefs that shape how you see yourself and the world around you.

Often, though, these beliefs are "self-limiting." They hold you back from achieving your goals and cut you off from enchanting possibilities for the future. Examples include: *I'll never be fit* or *It's in my DNA to be overweight* or *I'll never be successful* or *I'm not smart enough.*

Some aren't even your personal beliefs at all. They're passed down to you through family legacy or someone else's opinion of what you should believe, or based on past experiences, negative feedback from friends or associates, or even your own imagination.

There Is No Substitute for Authentic Human Connection

Here's where we focus on spiritual health—finding your purpose and connecting passionately with something bigger than yourself that gives your life meaning. Whether it's through religion, meditation, a special cause you support, or your work, spiritual health provides a sense of inner peace and helps you feel that you're part of a much bigger picture.

Spirituality is very tied to our fifth strategy—Connect—because you are committing to a community of people who believe what you believe. If you're in a dark place, the connection of joining a gym might pull you out of it.

That's because group exercise can be spiritual for many people! They gather with a community that gives them a ritual to perform together. You know who will be leading the workout; you can anticipate and feel the energy. You know you'll recognize familiar faces. You can congregate to actively socialize and celebrate with like-minded people—and as for many traditional spiritual practices, you'll also feel a deep sense of accomplishment when done. The shared experience of a hard-core workout brings participants closer together.

Also, moving with and around other highly motivated people not only releases a healthy dose of oxytocin but also challenges you to push the very edge of your fitness—and achieve personal excellence. As we know, this can be the big separator from being good to excellent.

Whatever its personal meaning to you, spirituality is rooted in faith—which is simply knowing that something greater than yourself exists even if it isn't physically there. With faith comes passion, purpose, and meaning.

Passion is an intense feeling derived from discovering your purpose and dedicating your life to the cause. The responsibility we bear in pursuit of this purpose gives our life meaning. When we train people to be Burn trainers, we always tell them that the first requirement to being an exceptional trainer is to be passionate about what they're doing. This works for anything in life. Most people will remember only 10 percent of what you say, but they will always remember how you made them feel. This feeling comes from your passion.

Passion is what gives you purpose—the force that gets you moving forward with what you want to create in your life. As a husband-and-wife team, our purpose became clear after we realized that fitness was our passion. We set out to positively affect as many people as we could, using our combined experiences in fitness, nutrition, and psychology—to found Burn Boot Camp. It was a fulfillment we had never experienced in our prior jobs—baseball and food marketing—and we just fell in love with helping and training people.

You see, we developed a strong sense of purpose. We figured out what we wanted, why we wanted it, and how we planned to achieve it. Along the way, we were willing to do hard things in order to pursue our purpose.

With passion and purpose, your life has meaning. You believe that you matter and that you matter to others. You feel that your life makes sense, you were put on the earth for a reason, and you're actively pursuing your goals. People who feel that their lives are meaningful tend to be happier and healthier.

The Believe strategy is involved in everything you do—and involved in every other strategy in this book. In Chapter 7, we'll show you how to implement it. For now, though, evaluate your time and be willing to make adjustments in the physical, mental, emotional, and spiritual realms of your life.

CHAPTER 3
STRATEGY #3: NOURISH

W E ALL GET ONE "AT BAT," ONE SWING AT LIFE. DO YOU WANT TO SPEND yours in fear, doubt, and shame? Or do you want to live a life of overcoming all obstacles? These are questions Kellie asked herself as she moved into a new phase of her life.

Kellie was active all her life—a former college athlete, then a personal trainer and a physical education teacher in elementary school. Then life hit. She was a stay-at-home mom to four children for ten years. Like most moms, Kellie put herself on the back burner. "I assumed my season of pursuing my passions for fitness had passed," she said. "As grateful as I am for those years, I had lost who I was in the thick of raising babies."

Kellie was no longer living in a body she recognized either, the combined result of three C-sections, a miscarriage, and the stress of a drawn-out, five-year adoption process. She was ashamed of her body and doubted that she could ever regain the strength and health of her youth. Although she ran 35 to 40 miles a week, Kellie's relationship with food was holding her back. No matter how long or hard she ran, she continued to put on weight and was low on energy because of poor food choices.

In November 2020, Kellie decided she needed a change and joined one of our camps in Springdale, Arkansas. "I was nervous and clung to the back row. But I was hooked after my first camp and instantly felt welcomed by everyone. I gradually started feeling like an athlete again. That confidence came back. It was a feeling I thought I'd never have again."

For Kellie, what she needed most of all was nutrition guidance. "Nutrition was never on my radar because the thought of how hard it would be to eat right overwhelmed me, especially while trying to feed a big family. I found the Burn meal plan to be a critical component to my success."

At the beginning of 2021, Kellie began to really look at her eating habits, making food swaps and learning to fuel her body properly, with a focus on getting stronger.

I desperately want my kids to have a healthy relationship with food, and I knew learning that at home is the best way to accomplish that. I took each day as an opportunity to improve my health, so they could see it in action. Every day I ate well was a victory that moved me that much closer to my goal. I shifted my thinking to Burn's idea of "one small win at a time." And eventually, I turned those small wins into a winning streak of long-term changes.

Kellie walked through the doors, looking for a new way to work out, but found much more: a supportive community, discipline, and a new way to eat. She's back to her former athletic self too, and more. Kellie is now certified in nutrition and is a strength and conditioning coach at a local high school. And she's passionate about all of it.

"My experience has been such a blessing, and it's so fun," she said. "I feel like I'm on a team again. And I know how great it feels to be pushed out of your comfort zone."

She added, "None of my accomplishments or titles define me. The real blessing is that I'm living in a body that is thriving, physically and mentally. It's not about perfection and impossible standards; it's about living a life I love for as long as possible."

Yes, Kellie got back into shape, but she learned that who she was becoming was FAR more important than how she looked. It was what she gained along her journey that was most important to her—a more positive spin on eating and exercising, and an appreciation for the miracle that is her body.

Here's where nutrition enters the picture, but from a different direction. For human beings, food is never just food. Food is intricately bound up in our relationships and social life. Food brings family and friends together. Food is a coping mechanism for feeling upset. Food is pleasurable to our palates.

We tend to forget, however, that food's primary purpose isn't to simply taste good and fill our stomach, or even to be manipulated for weight loss. Food is fuel. It gives us the physical and mental energy to go about our lives and helps us perform at our best. Once you connect your food with gaining energy rather than with losing weight, the game changes. It's all about energy!

Although there's nothing wrong with enjoying how your food tastes, or celebrating with food, our society never adopted the mindset that food is fuel, and we think this is a huge mistake. This mistargeted perspective is a massive part of why there is such an obesity epidemic around the world. To successfully become healthy, it's essential to change your mindset and see food as fuel.

This is what our Nourish strategy is all about: changing your mindset around food. Once you grasp this, you'll naturally get in shape in a sustainable way and be overflowing with energy. Please pause for a moment to let this soak in!

The Nourish strategy is also based on using high-quality, nutritious food to create inner strength, which (you now understand) leads to outer strength, in the same way that demanding **workouts** produce the same results. **The food you eat is *powerful*. It is the regulator of your physiology. It dramatically affects how you feel and how you perform.**

Many people don't get this. As a consequence, they're walking around feeling just "okay." That's not normal. You should feel great! And the way to feel great is through demanding workouts and high-quality foods—foods that maximize your health and quality of life. From your energy, your mood, your skin, to your performance, it all starts with what's on the end of your fork.

Let's be honest: we know you know how to diet; now let us teach you how to eat.

THE NOURISH STRATEGY HAS NOTHING TO DO WITH DIETING.

This strategy frees you from the "diet mentality," a self-destructive pattern of thinking and behaving. When you eat to "lose weight," you generally don't consider fuel or nourishment. You're doing the opposite—cutting nutrients like carbs or fat, along with calories. You're focused on what you can't eat or what you should or should not eat. Food as fuel isn't even on the radar.

It's clear that dieting is outdated and doesn't work. Aren't you sick of dieting, anyway? Everyone we talk to is sick of it and exhausted from the pop culture "diet whiplash," in which you get jerked around from one diet to the next. Dieting is a billion-dollar enterprise, and because it rarely works permanently, it comes with a ready supply of repeat customers. Statistics show that people are likely to regain the pounds they shed—and then gain a few more!

Instead of dieting, you'll learn to eat based on what nourishes your body, which is more about how food makes you feel, physically and mentally. A plan of whole foods, close to nature, mostly plants with a healthy dose of protein, is optimum for outstanding health.

If you nourish your body like this, you don't even need to worry so much about your food decisions—no obsessing over refined carbs, sugar, trans fat or saturated fat, or salt, for example. Focus on supporting your body with real food, and your weight and other food-related issues take care of themselves.

THE NOURISH STRATEGY BUILDS PHYSICAL HEALTH AND PREVENTS DISEASE.

Think about this for a moment: You can have all the money you'll ever need. You can own fabulous homes and expensive cars. You can have the best family and kids in the world. You can be at the top of your game in your career. But if you were sick with some disabling disease, none of it would matter at all. You'd give it all up in a second to have your health back, wouldn't you?

Of course, you would! This is where nourishing yourself with high-quality food is a must, along with physical activity. The decision to eat the right foods can put an end to taking pills, suffering chronic headaches and gut problems, frequent infections from flu and colds, dealing with weight ups and downs, and more—and help you thrive every single day.

We know, too, that certain eating patterns help lower your risk for particular diseases. For example, the recommendations for reducing the risk of dementia emphasize vegetables, fruits, seafood, legumes, and nuts. The same foods are the main dietary elements that have proved most beneficial in preventing or treating other serious diseases, from heart disease to cancer to diabetes.

Proper nourishment is not complicated, and it doesn't have to be grandiose. Eat foods that come from the earth, and don't overeat. It's that simple.

THE NOURISH STRATEGY EMPHASIZES CLEAN FUEL FOR EXERCISE AND DAILY ACTIVITIES.

To train hard, eat for fuel and nourishment. It gives you the energy to do an extra rep each workout, and that translates into greater fitness. It boosts and sustains your energy levels, keeps you focused on tasks at hand, powers your daily activities, builds muscle, supplies you with vital nutrients, and so much more. If you eat nutrient-rich, minimally processed foods rather than junk food, you'll perform better during exercise and, really, throughout your day. That's the magic of food as nourishment.

Imagine your body as your car. Quality food is the fuel required to start the engine and drive off. So fuel your body with high-octane nutrients to ensure you feel and perform at your best.

THE NOURISH STRATEGY BOOSTS YOUR BRAINPOWER.

Do you realize that your brain is always "on"? It processes thoughts, regulates your breathing and heartbeat, controls hunger and appetite, and coordinates how you move. It's on the job 24/7, even while you're asleep. To stay on top of that job, your brain requires a steady supply of fuel from food and the nutrients in that food.

Eat natural, whole foods packed with vitamins, minerals, and antioxidants, and you'll nourish your brain and protect it from "oxidative stress." This refers to the "waste" (cell-damaging free radicals) generated as your body consumes oxygen.

If you eat junk food loaded with sugar, additives, preservatives, and other toxins, those substances reach the brain, and it has trouble flushing them out. Sugar is a real problem and can cause inflammation. Excess sugar in the diet interferes with the body's ability to properly use insulin. This hormone is responsible for escorting blood sugar inside cells to be burned for energy. When insulin can't do this job, sugar builds up, causing inflammation in the brain—which can lead to mental decline.

When your brain is operating on clean fuel, you'll perform better on your job too. Try this with us: Recall your most productive workday recently. Now ask yourself: On that day, what did you eat for lunch?

When we think about what gets us ahead in our careers, food rarely comes to mind. Yet for those of us working hard to succeed, food is extremely important because it affects our productivity.

Here's why: Just about everything we eat is broken down into glucose (blood sugar), which energizes our brain to remain alert. When glucose is in short supply, we have a tough time staying focused. In fact, our attention span can get shorter than that of a goldfish, which is nine seconds.

Scientists now assert that we humans generally lose concentration after eight seconds!

So far, pretty clear. Now here's the part we don't think about: Some foods, such as white bread, candy and other sweets, any processed food, and soda, are converted into glucose fast. We get a burst of energy. This is followed by a quick, sharp drop in blood sugar, making us groggy. Unhealthy lunch options like these won't boost our productivity!

So, what should you do? The important move is to nourish yourself with whole foods (no processed or fast foods) at lunchtime. We're talking about salads, lean proteins like chicken or tuna, nuts, or a sandwich made with whole grains or sprouted bread. Foods like these maintain your glucose at a more consistent level and provide you with the mental energy to stay on top of your game.

THE NOURISH STRATEGY CREATES INNER STRENGTH.

The best part? Great food makes you feel great mentally. When you feel great, you're more productive. When you're more productive, you have more pride. When you have more pride, your confidence grows. And when your confidence grows, you are unstoppable.

We're talking about the mood-boosting advantages of nourishing yourself well. Healthy choices like fruits, vegetables, whole grains, and lean proteins can ease depression, stabilize your mood, and keep you out of the stress-eating zone where it feels like only a big ice cream sundae will save the day.

In research appearing in the *American Journal of Psychiatry* in 2010, investigators analyzed the meal patterns of 1,046 women aged twenty to ninety-three. They discovered that those who followed a healthy diet, centering on vegetables, fruits, fish, lean meat, and whole grains, were less likely to suffer depression and anxiety than those who followed a Western diet loaded with refined grains, sugar, fried foods, and junk food. No wonder! The Western way of eating lacks such nutrients as vitamins, minerals, and healthy fats—all of which support healthy function and mood.

Nutritious food is a mood booster!

What Foods Can I Eat to Boost My Mood?

Quite a few! Take a look.

Fruits and vegetables. You know the wise, familiar maxim "An apple a day keeps the doctor away." Well, apples and other plant foods may keep the psychiatrist away too. Eating fruits and veggies on a regular basis has been correlated with higher levels of happiness and less depression.

Omega-3 fatty acids. This is the super-healthy stuff found in such foods as fish, nuts, and nut oils. A good supply of omega-3 fatty acids in the diet helps alleviate depression.

Fermented foods. These include cultured milk, tempeh, kimchi, yogurt, kombucha, and sauerkraut. Fermentation is a process by which certain nutrients are broken down to make the food more digestible. During the fermentation, probiotics are created. These are friendly, live microorganisms that support a healthy gut and may increase levels of the mood-boosting brain chemical serotonin.

Bananas. This delicious fruit is packed with vitamin B_6, which helps manufacture feel-good brain chemicals like dopamine and serotonin.

Berries. These little fruits are loaded with antioxidants that may help protect brain cells and ease depression and other mood disorders.

Nuts and seeds. These plant-based proteins supply tryptophan, an amino acid that is a building block for mood-boosting serotonin.

Beans and lentils. Nutritional powerhouses, these plant foods are a rich source of B vitamins, known to boost mood. B vitamins increase levels of many regulating chemicals in the body.

Dark chocolate. Here's a treat with properties that also improve mood and even reduce tension. Choose real chocolate (dark is best), and enjoy it in moderation.

OKAY, WHAT'S IT GOING TO TAKE?

To live this strategy, it's going to require discipline and a new attitude toward food. Let go of what you did or thought yesterday. It's gone. It's time for a fresh start. Today is a new day, and tomorrow is another one—more chances to make the right choices, apply common sense when it comes to food selection, and change your overall psychology and mindset around food so you no longer have to rely upon willpower alone.

What you eat matters for every aspect of your life. If you want what high-quality food delivers, pay careful attention to a food's level of purity, and eat mostly foods that meet standards of unrefined freshness. Simply put, if it isn't created naturally by the earth, don't eat it. To stay the course with this strategy:

Nourishing Your Body Is Loving Your Body

Feeding your body with healthy, nutritious food is a form of self-love. Self-love means that you care about your own well-being and happiness, and you do everything you can to support your physical, mental, emotional, and spiritual growth. When you love yourself, you put yourself first, believe you are important, and show yourself kindness and self-compassion.

Once you internalize the truth that food is fuel, you'll find it easier to love yourself with nutritious foods. Start by connecting with the idea that you deserve to feel good in your body; then love your body by providing it with excellent nutrition that makes you feel amazing from the inside out.

Morgan learned about nourishment and self-love the hard way. As she tells it:

My first fitness role model was my mother. I distinctly remember the VCR bringing Jane Fonda into our living room, clad in a leotard and leg warmers, doing her leg lifts and step aerobics. Mom's meal afterward was another grapefruit. Becoming as thin as you could be was the goal. Whittle it away, shrink it down, restrict, deny.

In my twenties, I found competitive bodybuilding. The sport intrigued me because I was a three-sport athlete in high school and loved to compete. But bodybuilding required crazy, unhealthy practices to slash body fat to extremely low percentages. I fasted. I ate bland chicken breasts. I took appetite suppressants. I wore my body down with hours of conditioning and strength training every day. When I wasn't training obsessively, I constantly compared my body to [that of] other female bodybuilders and concluded that I did not measure up or look as good. I began to hate my body and everything about it, all because I had such a poor relationship with food and exercise.

Not only did I begin to notice my energy and physical health declining rapidly, but so was my mental health. I didn't feel worthy, good enough, strong enough, or sexy enough. I was constantly critiquing my body. I was miserable.

One night, I looked at myself in the mirror. Staring back at me were sunken cheeks, a pasty complexion, and a worn-out look. I knew that what I was doing was destroying my body. And although there was no way I could train harder or cut more body fat, every time I looked in the mirror, I only saw my flaws. I only saw someone who wouldn't place in the top three. It was the beginning of body dysmorphia and a scary downward spiral. "Why the hell am I doing this?" I asked myself tearfully. "This isn't me."

I quit competitive bodybuilding then and there. Realizing that my food choices could make or break my health was a transformative decision that taught me the importance of self-love. Ultimately, I forgave myself and accepted my body and appearance, the first step toward fixing my relationship with food.

After that happened, I found my purpose; to be a leader in the fitness profession to help other women accept and love their bodies.

Accept yourself as you are right now. Embrace and love your body. It is the most amazing thing you will ever own. Express that love by eating healthy food for your body and staying active. Show your body love. You deserve it.

STOP TELLING YOURSELF FOOD LIES.

Remember, we have more daily internal conversations with ourselves than all conversations with friends, family, and coworkers combined. We speak to others carefully and with respect because we want to maintain strong relationships with them. But how do we speak to ourselves? Totally differently—and usually without much self-respect at all! In fact, we tell ourselves a lot of negative lies about ourselves! In working with members, we've listened to many lies they tell themselves that block their fitness and nutritional success. Here are some of the biggest we've heard.

I'm fat.

You're not fat; you may have fat. You also have fingernails. You're not a fingernail. You also have armpits, but you're not an armpit. You also have eyelids; you are not an eyelid.

Calling yourself fat is not healthy. If you do this long enough, you might even get fat. One study found that women who think they are overweight are more likely to put on weight in the long run, even if they were not overweight to begin with.

Why do any of us call ourselves fat, anyway? We fling the word around like it's no big deal when, in fact, it is. When you go through the day saying "I am fat," expect bad choices to dog you. We encourage the use of phrases like "I am healthy," "I am strong," "I am courageous," "I am joyful," and "I am fulfilled." These "I am" transformations in your language have a tremendous impact on how you perceive your life and how you change positively as a result. Using "I am" in this context may seem like a small, subtle thing to do, but we've seen it radically transform thousands of lives.

I can't eat that food.

Imagine you're eating exceptionally cleanly and working on improving your health and performance. You're finishing a nice meal at your favorite restaurant. Your server clears the plates and says, "You know, we have a new, delicious chocolate cheesecake on our dessert menu. Would you like to try it?"

What's running through your mind? Are you thinking: "I can't eat cheesecake"? Or are you thinking: "I don't eat cheesecake"?

There's a distinct psychological difference in these two mindsets. And if there's one important lesson from psychology, subtle differences in your self-talk have an enormously powerful impact on your thoughts, feelings, and actions.

In the above example, "I don't" expresses a choice. It's empowering, and a wonderful demonstration of your free will. "I can't" is not technically a choice. Rather, it's a restraint you're imposing on yourself. So, thinking or saying "I can't" restricts your personal power, control, and accountability.

The dramatic difference between these two phrases has even been researched. In one study, twenty adult women who were focused on hitting their health and fitness goals were instructed to use the words *I don't* or *I can't* when tempted to cheat (for example, skip their workout or grab a candy bar).

Which strategy worked best? You guessed it: by the study's end, eight of the ten women who employed the *I don't* language were able to better hold off on temptations, plus achieve their goals with greater success. Those using *I can't* didn't fare so well. So every time you catch yourself about to think or say: *I can't have this*, substitute *No, I don't want this*, instead.

I'm always hungry, or starving.

Hunger—uncomfortable? Yes. Annoying? Maybe. Feeling hungry forever? Not possible. The truth is, hunger usually passes. When you convince yourself that your hunger is nothing more than a temporary feeling of minor discomfort, you're far more likely to make healthy choices.

People will also say, "I am so starving, I could eat a cow!" Really? You're starving? Using the term "starving" implies that you're suffering or dying from hunger. Isn't it more appropriate to say "I'm just a little bit hungry"?

We tend to use words, without realizing it, that intensify our emotions. The language we use creates the meaning of what we're saying. The meaning of what we're saying dictates the emotions we feel. The emotions we feel control the actions we take. The actions we take control the outcome of our lives. Did you follow that? Let's break it down with an example.

When you say, "I'm starving," you're talking yourself into a state of deprivation. A common emotion connected to deprivation is suffering. When you believe you're suffering from starvation, you'll do whatever it takes to get your hands on as much food as possible in fear that you may not eat again. When you do this repeatedly, you're risking weight gain, even obesity, which ultimately leads to a life of lethargy, low energy, poor confidence, and low self-esteem.

Sometimes you're truly hungry, and other times, you think you're hungry. Recall a time when you said "I'm starving," and then you received an important phone call or text. What happened? Your new focus took you away from the thought of eating, and you began to focus on something more important. Before you knew it, the urge to eat passed.

What happened? You had experienced a false hunger cue. Be on the lookout for these. When you feel hungry, either preoccupy yourself with something else and let the urge pass, or grab a healthy snack of fruit, veggies, or nuts.

I've failed so many times before, I'll fail again.

Do you habitually beat yourself up over going off a diet and declaring yourself a hopeless cause?

Watch out! This attitude creates unhelpful feelings like shame, guilt, and resentment, and can lead to unproductive behavior like poor eating or lack of exercise.

Just because you fail doesn't mean you're a failure. In fact, with every failure you learn what doesn't work, so you can figure out what does. In that way, failure is just another stepping stone to success.

If you've had a setback, remind yourself of the successes you have had in other areas of your life. Tell yourself something like *"I've overcome tough things before. I can do it again."*

When our children were very small, we slipped up in our nutrition as parents. Yes, we made sure our kids got all the protein, vitamins, and minerals they needed. But although we knew how to eat nutritiously, we just weren't doing it ourselves. We'd get so exhausted at times that we'd order takeout, while our children got the healthy stuff. But once the kids got older, we said, "Enough is enough. We're going back to what we know best—healthy eating."

Recalling times when you've bounced back equips you with the knowledge, tools, and talents that worked for you before—and can now be used to succeed. How you handle failure proves that you're tougher than you think, and you can handle more than you know.

PRACTICE FOOD AWARENESS.

The food we eat is made up of calories, which are units of energy for our body. Along with oxygen, they are what keeps our body fueled and functioning. Every calorie is composed of three macronutrients—protein, carbohydrates, and fats. These units of energy enter our body, determine our internal health, and play a role in our weight and level of body fat—a process called "energy balance."

This process is especially important in conquering overweight and obesity—two conditions that gravely affect physical and mental health. To overcome or prevent them, you must put your body in a calorie deficit. If this statement were merely an opinion, we could see alternate ways to argue it, but it's a scientific fact. If you want to shed pounds and burn body fat, you must expend more calories (energy) than you consume. No matter what the diet—keto, Paleo, Atkins, low fat, high protein, and others—for you to lose body fat naturally, it has to create a calorie deficit. Nothing works if you overconsume calories.

Once your body's energy needs are met, extra calories are packed away for future use—some in your muscles as glycogen, and some stored in fat tissue. Thus, eating more calories than you burn may promote weight gain, whereas eating fewer than you need triggers weight loss. Calorie balance is critically important to weight management.

Let's face it, counting calories is no fun. We don't like it either, but you don't have to like everything that's good for you. So what we teach is "calorie accountability," a more intuitive approach to nourishment.

To become food aware:

Learn your food. Our goal is to educate you until you no longer need us! Refreshing to hear fitness professionals saying that, isn't it? We believe an educated person is an empowered person—and we want to empower you as well.

The way that you "learn your food" is to track your calories and nutrients, using an app to log in your meals. If you're new to this, spend a month tracking and logging. You don't have to make it a career path, though! After that, you can log one to two days a week just to stay sharp and on top of your calorie accountability. Eventually, you'll be so knowledgeable about food that that you can "eyeball" your calories and macros.

Logging itself isn't the trick, though. What moves the needle for your nutritional knowledge is the curiosity you bring to the act of logging. You've got to take the time to initially study your logs and be hungry to learn! Knowledge is power. Once you know what you're eating and how nutritious it is, you're much more likely to stay the course.

Plan your food. Anticipation is power, and the more you plan your menus, the more you'll succeed. The "whoops, I forgot about food" moments during the middle of the workday are minimized when you're prepared in advance. On the road, we look at our schedule ahead of time and plan to make stops at certain Whole Foods or Chipotle, or other markets or restaurants that serve healthy food.

Love your food. With calorie accountability, we believe you can really love healthy food! Most of us know that habitually scarfing down fast food, processed food, or sugary snacks is not the best food decision, and for many, may be unhealthy habits. To break habits like this:

- Become aware of, and acknowledge, an unhealthy eating habit. (You can't change negative behaviors unless you identify them first.)
- Replace it with a desirable behavior.
- Reinforce the desirable behavior with self-love.

A real-world example might be this: You come home from work and habitually dive into a box of cookies, devouring a bunch of them. Your brain begins to develop a well-trodden neural pathway to cookie-eating.

Replace that behavior by eating a handful of sweet, juicy grapes every day. Congratulate and love yourself for your better choice. Keep making these choices. You can have some cookies if you really want some. But chances are, you'll start feeling so good about resisting the cookies that your brain associates not eating them with a pleasurable experience. Your brain no longer considers a cookie to be a better reward than grapes.

SHOOT FOR SMALL WINS.

We'll show you how to make just five small changes in your eating habits: eat 100 grams of protein a day, remove added sugar, increase your fluid intake, control your alcohol consumption, and actively practice calorie accountability.

We call these "small wins" (see Chapter 8) and they lead to big, lasting change. You can't develop great health habits overnight. Lasting change requires a gradual approach. If you try to bite off more than you can chew (pun intended!)—like tackling big, dramatic lifestyle changes—chances are you'll get discouraged and feel defeated. And discouragement and defeat are no longer options.

Healthy nutrition has been daunting to you in the past because you've had poor strategies. We've tried all the fads too. Nothing works like educating yourself and realizing that "diet life" consists of hype and unattainable promises. You must eat the right food to have the productive output you want, and there are no other options. Get ready to start *thinking* about food differently.

FOLLOW OUR BURN 10-MINUTE MEAL PLAN.

One of the best ways to be successful, plus stay food aware, is to incorporate our meal-planning process into your lifestyle. The way it works is simple. The plan (see Chapter 8) is made up of five calorie-accountable meals and snacks. Each day, you choose from among fifty recipes that take no longer than ten minutes to prepare. You then mix and match your breakfasts, lunches, dinners, and snacks into a daily plan that meets your caloric requirement. All the calories, protein, carbohydrates, and fat are already calculated for you.

Another important part of the process involves meal preparation. We'll show you how to set aside three hours a week to execute this, including ninety minutes to shop and ninety minutes to prepare. Example: Cook your protein, and while that's cooking, prepare three sides. This will make three meals. When done, place them in glassware and reheat prior to meals. Do this twice a week, on Sundays or Wednesdays—and voilà, you are set for the week.

Most people think they need to deploy complex plans. No! Complexity is the enemy of execution. We value easy executing—so we've made all of this a breeze for you.

Think of the Nourish strategy as a new mindset, and this will be the last time you have to struggle with food issues—no more starting over with the latest fad diet! Believe that you can eat nutritiously and still enjoy an *exciting adventure with food* without hard-core, restrictive rules. With this strategy, you'll cement **a lifelong commitment to healthy nutrition, with changes to your way of eating you'll want to keep forever.**

CHAPTER 4

STRATEGY #4: ACHIEVE

ANCER, COVID-19, A BROKEN MARRIAGE. THESE TRAGEDIES HIT Cynthia, from our Fayetteville, Georgia, camp, all in a row, and it's a wonder how she coped. But she not only coped, she got through them. Cynthia was focused and goal-oriented, which allowed her to overcome these challenges. Hers is a story of how we can let tragedy either destroy us and make us bitter or make us stronger.

Cynthia had always been athletic, a self-professed workout junkie. Even after the pandemic hit in 2020, she continued her workouts faithfully at home and on Zoom. That same year, her husband took a job in South Carolina and moved the family to a small, isolated community. The marriage was already failing; the move did not help. She found herself in a relationship where she had given up her own ambitions and passions, which took her confidence and self-worth with it. She realized she was in a partnership that was working for the good of one.

Then, in June 2021, Cynthia received devastating news that shook her world.

"I was diagnosed with breast cancer. My world shattered. I went from biopsy to surgery to chemo very quickly," she recalled. "The chemo crushed my body for two months. I was nauseous and tired all the time. I lost all my strength. My body was fully drained, and I was in constant pain. I was fighting for my life every single day."

During this time, Cynthia separated from her husband. Medical bills piled up. Physically, mentally, and emotionally, she felt that she was in an unyielding storm. Unbelievably, she kept her focus on fitness. She continued to work out but used exercise modifications her trainers put together for her. She found solace in two places: her loving family and her friends at her gym. They became her pillars of strength, reminding her of the vibrant life that was waiting for her beyond the shadows of cancer and heartbreak. At one very low point, she realized she didn't have the money to afford her membership, her lifeline. That's when another member stepped in and paid for a full year of workouts on her behalf.

At the beginning of 2023, Cynthia entered one of our Burn Boot Camp challenges, a friendly competition to help members realize how capable they are of exceeding their fitness expectations. She stuck with it. She did not once give up on her workouts or on herself.

"Life was very different then. But I did not get this far to throw in the towel. Even baby steps moved me forward. Sure, the challenge was hard, but my Burn sisters supported me and helped me complete it. It was the most exhilarating experience. At that moment, I knew I was going to make it."

Cynthia stayed focused on achieving one goal—returning to the strength she had in 2020. As her body healed, her heart also healed from the pain of her failed marriage. She realized how much of her independence she had given up to prioritize her husband's happiness. She now had the ability to make choices that aligned with her goals, chart her own path, and define her worth on her terms. "The workouts kept me sane, and I got physically stronger all the time. It has been a roller coaster, and I'm still dealing with medical bills. But God has me, and I feel His hand on me. And my gym has kept me centered. It became my anchor and solidified my love for my Burn community. I am where I am physically and mentally because of my work-outs and the trainers and members who support me every day."

Cynthia gave herself another day, another chance. She found cour-age, strength, and love from those around her, and amazing things happened.

Have you ever wondered what the difference is between people who seem to succeed at everything versus those who fail and give up? Why do some people like Cynthia hang in there and reach their goals, yet others don't even try? We've asked ourselves these questions for years, and we've finally got the answer.

It's simple. Successful people know exactly what they want and why they want it, and they spend every waking minute going after it. They have a clearly defined sense of direction. They've discovered an enchant-ing purpose and view success as their only option. They believe in achiev-ing positive results so strongly that they become unstoppable. They overcome every obstacle with determination so fierce that nothing holds them back.

Wouldn't you like to join those ranks?

You can! Success comes down to knowing how to set the right goals, prioritize the steps to achieve them, and adhere to the plan.

Goals give direction to your life, a road to travel on. Yet a lot of people struggle with setting them. Some may have already given up. Others are just letting the whole thing slide. Still others set goals aimlessly or without conviction, which leaves them uncertain about whether they will ever achieve their goal. Their motivation lasts for only a few weeks, and then they revert to their old habits. At some point, they deal with the frustra-tion of having to start over—and so begins a crazy cycle of starting and stopping and never reaching any goal.

Also, many people confuse goals with outcomes. Have you ever had a goal like "I want to drop 15 pounds" or "I need to switch jobs," and six months later, you're still in the exact same situation as when you started? Why?

Because things like "lose 15 pounds" and "switch jobs" aren't *good enough* goals, they're outcomes. Sure, they're okay to want, but as goals, they're worthless. In fact, they can actually block you from getting what you want, if things don't go your way. You end up feeling defeated—which is why you've repeatedly had to start over throughout your life.

Other people set goals that are too low, or they don't even bother to set them. A goal that's too low is an indication you're scared. Not setting them at all is a sign that you're currently unmotivated.

Setting the right goals is a necessary step on the road to change. And for many of us, it can be exhilarating. It's a way of telling yourself what's important to you and committing energy to it.

You're capable of amazing things. There's nothing that is impossible, out of reach, or too outrageous to get. Do you want to open your own business or go back to school? Would you like to be independently wealthy? Do you want to be a better parent or have a more loving, supportive relationship? Do you want to lose body fat and feel more confident? How about feeling more satisfied and at peace?

The good news is that you can have all this and more. We have a guaranteed GPS—a directional guide—for successful living, one that absolutely works.

That GPS is the Achieve strategy. It helps you clarify your dreams, start doing what you want, and make things happen in your life.

When you're clear about what you want and you develop a vision for your life, amazing things start happening because you are doing what you love and following your heart. More opportunities show up, doors open, and all sorts of wonderful things come your way.

Here's how the Achieve strategy works.

THE ACHIEVE STRATEGY TEACHES YOU HOW TO SET "NORTH STAR GOALS."

A North Star goal is a guiding compass for every decision you make and every step you take. It is not pragmatic, short-term, or utilitarian like losing

20 pounds or competing in the New York City Marathon, but rather an overarching life goal of how you want to live your life.

There are two driving forces behind North Star goals. The first is love. Love is the oxygen of life. We will go to great lengths physically, mentally, emotionally, and spiritually to protect the relationships in our lives.

Supported by numerous studies, love activates the parts of the brain that control our drive to achieve goals. When we love, we're motivated to please those we care about. In doing so, the brain churns out dopamine— a neurotransmitter vital to reward-motivated behavior—as well as oxytocin, the bonding hormone. Love makes you want to be a better person for those you love.

What would you do if someone you love became extremely ill, and the only way to save them was to come up with $50,000 for some lifesaving procedure? Certainly, you'd find a way to raise the money. After all, your love for them is so strong that *not* raising the money would not be an option. How creative would you get? Wouldn't you go to great lengths to save them?

Of course you would! When a loss of love is on the line, you'll do whatever is necessary to maintain the connection.

The second driving force behind a North Star goal is a personally motivating vision. It's been said that you need to "see it to be it." So imagine your ideal life in ten to twenty years, where you are enjoying feeling accomplished and successful.

Ask yourself: What needs to happen in the coming months and years for me to feel truly successful? What must I accomplish? What do I really want to transform? Why do I want to really transform? What does success look like for me?

Then dream of the person you want to be and the life you want. It's not so much how wealthy or powerful or famous your future self might be—but about the life you will lead and how you will make a difference, leaving the world a better and more beautiful place.

Then concentrate on what you'll do to get there and the joy you'll gain from the positive journey of creating value and loving others along the way. Each day, consider what you will do with your health, in your work, with your mental and emotional actions, your spiritual life, and your relationships to keep you going forward. Your vision helps you control the direction you move toward. From that, you create the steps to get there. And when you start working on them, you get clarity and purpose. Finally, your vision becomes reality. (More on visualization in Chapter 9.)

You'll know you've created an effective North Star goal when the mere thought of it leaves you feeling excited, energized, and motivated to make it a reality.

Motivation Is Push and Pull

There are two forces moving you to action: push goals and pull goals. Pull goals are something you've imagined that you're running toward (your vision of the future). They are pulling you forward, creating momentum because they are exciting. An example is being healthy and happy when your granddaughter is born or living until one hundred in amazing health.

Push goals are something you've experienced in the past that was super painful—a place you never want to be again. You're pushing away from this, but toward your goal. In our family, for example, we want to create a life for our children in which they have everything they need and are safe from danger. We don't want them growing up like we did (especially Devan). Another example of a push goal: "I don't want to be overweight anymore; I'm tired of feeling tired and weak. I don't want to be like my parents and miss out on my kid's childhood." Push goals always have to do with something in the past that you don't like.

The idea is that "future" and "past" experiences are both very valuable. We either move away from something we don't want (a push goal) or toward something we do want (a pull goal). When we do both, this is a superpower.

We need both push and pull goals to get us where we want to be and maximize the probability of success.

THE ACHIEVE STRATEGY INVOLVES SMALL, ACTIONABLE WINS.

After setting your North Star goals, you'll want to "reverse engineer" them. This involves breaking your North Star goal down into smaller, more manageable pieces—say, the next five to ten moves you make to get you there. You work back from the North Star goal to figure out what you need to stop, what you need to start, and what action to take daily or weekly to accomplish your North Star goal. Instead of trying to do everything at once, you tackle a little bit one day at a time, make decisions that move you toward your goal, and turn away from things that don't.

For instance, if you want to become a teacher, you'll need to go to college, make good grades, graduate from college with a teaching degree, gain any appropriate work experience—and then be hired for a teaching job.

It is not what you do once in a while that determines your success. It's what you do every day. Success is not a onetime action, but it is continuous progress through actionable moves that lead you to the outcome you want.

These moves are "small wins," which we discussed in Chapter 3.

Small wins are anything you accomplish that are aligned with your goals. They might be associated with your work, relationships, health, habits, and so forth. Examples of small wins are cutting refined sugar out of your diet, finishing a workout, putting extra money in savings, or completing a project.

Small wins are powerful confidence builders. When you're faced with failure, it's easy to lose your self-confidence and self-esteem. But did you know that accomplishing small wins can do the opposite—ramp up your self-esteem and confidence?

When you set up your day to get small wins, you'll have a positive day, every day. You feel productive, and you get done little tedious jobs that you may have otherwise put off if you weren't in the mood. You'll feel engaged, happy, and worthy. This creates a positive feedback loop. The more small wins you have, the more motivated you'll be to keep pursuing your goals. Before you know it, you've proved to yourself that you can

actually get things done, even if you thought small processes were insignif-
icant and wouldn't help you reach your outcomes.

As such, you're activating the magic of momentum. It's the concept of
falling forward. Leaning into our failures or challenges and using them as
a learning tool to continue growing. It's like stumbling through a maze
in the dark, where even your missteps are a chance to inch closer to your
goals.

Momentum holds one of the greatest factors of success: continuous
progress toward extraordinary success in life.

THE ACHIEVE STRATEGY APPLIES TO EVERY AREA OF YOUR LIFE.

We feel that there are eight categories of personal success. If you aren't
satisfied with some of these areas, the Achieve strategy steers you in a
positive direction.

Body. How do you want to feel after you get up in the morning? What
level of health or wellness do you want? How healthy do you want to be, or
how strong and fit do you want to feel?

These are questions to ask yourself to set the most important North
Star goal—the one that involves the most important thing you have,
your body. Taking care of your body improves longevity, prevents diseases,
improves mental and emotional health, and even brings financial benefits
(healthy people are more productive and prosperous). Without a healthy
body, you really have nothing.

Mind. Whatever you think about, you will become—which is why this
part of your life is so important. Mental health is the foundation of all you
do and how you feel—mainly because your thoughts become your behav-
ior and your behavior becomes your habits.

Emotions. What feelings do you want to carry through each day? More
zest for life? A deep sense of exhilaration? A feeling of inner peace? More
enthusiasm? Do you want to better regulate your emotions? Do you want
to be happier? Do you want to feel more contentment?

Emotions affect how you think and behave. They can compel you to take action, or be paralyzing and hold you back. Overall, they influence the decisions you make about your life, both large and small.

Spirit. Going through life can be very empty and dissatisfying without spiritual connection and support. Spirituality gives meaning to your life, helps you find purpose, and spares you from much unnecessary stress. It helps you understand the power of love in the world and how everything originates from that love. When you have spirituality, you feel a part of this loving energy and recognize that all you strive for comes from this place.

Relationships. What kind of people do you want to hang around with? What kind of a spouse, friend, parent, grandparent, sister, brother, father, or mother would you like to be? How do you want to make people feel?

Relationships are a vital element of a truly successful life. To achieve North Star goals in this area, you've got to take care of yourself first— which goes back to strategies 1 (Burn) and 3 (Nourish). We know that in our own lives, when we take care of ourselves first, we're happier and far less likely to react in anger and frustration and more likely to give love and joy. When we feel good and have clarity, we can love one another better and spend quality time every day with our family.

Give yourself the gift of loving yourself first, and you'll generate an abundance of happiness that will spill over not only into your intimate relationships but also into your work life.

Time. Time is your most precious asset, and it passes every single day. Once time is gone, you never get it back. You'll never be able to relieve this moment, be this age, or experience this season of life again. So, how are you going to use your time?

For one thing, stop telling yourself you don't have enough time. That's just another way of saying a goal isn't important enough for you—that it's not a priority. When you are your number one priority, you'll make time to be happy and healthy by default.

Lack of time is an illusion, anyway. We used to say, "We only have one hour. That's not enough time" or "Why aren't there more hours in the day?" Then we shifted our thinking (which goes back to the Believe strategy) to "We have an hour. How much can we get done?" or "How much can I accomplish in every hour of every day?" With just this simple change in thinking, our productivity went through the roof, and we had more time to spend with our kids.

Work. Do you look forward to your job? What level of fulfillment do you get from your job? Why are you there? Why are you doing what you're doing?

If you're like most people, you spend 75 percent of your waking existence working. So if you have a job, let's hope you love it and look forward to doing it! If you don't, there's a problem. You need to be engaged in work that brings you pleasure, fulfillment, and purpose. Work is too big a deal to not take seriously.

Personally speaking, we work fifteen to eighteen hours a day, every day. We haven't taken a lengthy vacation in years, but it's because we enjoy our work. We actually feel better at work than we do on vacation. If you love what you do and you're happy with your contribution to the world, it's part of who you are and it never feels like work.

We're not suggesting that working long hours and skipping vacations will make you happy. We're suggesting that you set goals for yourself that lead you to loving your work and following your passions.

Money. What role do you want money to play in your life? Do you want to be debt-free and achieve financial freedom? Do you want to save for retirement or an emergency fund? Do you want to learn more about investing? Do you need to budget more effectively? Do you want to donate more to charities? What do you want to be earning in five, ten, or twenty years? What talents can you use to get there?

These are important questions. For example, you might want to have a net worth of $3 million in the next five years or you want to retire at age fifty with X amount of dollars in investments. Then you can adopt North Star goals that will get you there.

OKAY, WHAT IS IT GOING TO TAKE?

Setting your goals and achieving them is a skill. And as with any other skills, you can train yourself to get good at it. Yes, you can become a pro at setting and achieving your goals—and ultimately be who and what you want from this moment on. Here's how.

Think Big

Remember what we said? Nothing is impossible!

Don't be paralyzed by huge goals. Putting big goals out into the universe points you toward success. We learned this the hard way!

In the very early days of our company, we had no clue about goal-setting or its benefits. We initially set a goal of opening five hundred locations, but how to get there? No idea, especially when our beginnings were so rocky.

It all began in 2012 in a parking lot behind a children's gymnastics facility on a blazing hot day in Charlotte, North Carolina. After moving to Charlotte, we spent ninety days searching for a spot to sublease so that we could lead group fitness classes (what we call camps), and the parking lot was the only available option. We signed up twenty-one people and bought $600 worth of used, rusty dumbbells.

Eight people showed up the first day, but no one else came by the end of the week. The endeavor was off to a shaky start and had to be turned around, or else we would continue to be broke.

With vision, our passion for health, and fierce determination, we promoted Burn, by doing a deep dive into social media, public relations, and content creation. After the local *Huntersville Herald* published an article titled "Ex Professional Baseball Player Trains Local Moms," the enterprise took off. Within two months, the parking lot was flooded with people.

Positive momentum continued, and more people showed up at our five parking lot gyms. Burn Boot Camp grew from zero-paying clients to one thousand paying members within twelve months. Then we flipped them all into brick-and-mortar facilities. Next, two people approached us to find out how Burn Boot Camps could be set up in other cities. We closed a deal with them, launched these facilities, and eventually converted them from licensing operations to franchises. By February 2017, Burn Boot Camp had become one of the fastest-growing franchises in the world, awarding over two hundred territories in our first eighteen months of business.

With this rapid success, we've set our vision to ten thousand units globally and being the largest fitness company in the world. Think big when there is no logical reason not to.

Be Specific

Your North Star goals should be so specific and clear that a first grader can understand them. That's why "I want to be fit" or "I want to be successful" fail the test. Everyone wants that stuff, but they're too generic. What does all that really mean? More to the point, there's no specific emotional attachment to the statement. If you want more money, ask for a dollar, and voilà, more money!

A North Star goal would state: "I want to be fit because I will feel confident, and my example will help my kids grow up with confidence." In the example at the start of this chapter, Cynthia was specific. She wanted to regain her strength so that she could live her life fully—physically, mentally, and emotionally.

The downfall for a lot of people is not being specific enough and getting exactly what they ask for. In other words, don't be someone who is wandering through life with no specific direction. Instead, be someone who stands out from the crowd and gets what they ask for.

The more specific your goals and the more you focus on them, the more your reticular activating system (RAS) will attract opportunities to make them happen. Align your thoughts with what you want and the life you desire—ask and you shall receive—and the RAS goes to work. It will present information on what it will take to accomplish your goals.

Record Your North Star Goals

When we give talks or deliver keynote speeches, we ask people, "How many of you have specific goals written down that you could show me if I asked you?" Usually, only about 10 percent of those in the room raise their hand.

North Star goals aren't real until they are written down on a piece of paper and stored next to your bed, and read, and reread every night and day. This keeps an emotional fire lit underneath your everyday actions.

Also, when you write down your North Star goals, describe them as if you've already achieved them. Why? Because your subconscious mind can't process a goal unless it's in the present tense. This confirms that your reticular activating system kicks in. When you know exactly what you want and you think about it constantly, read it daily, and talk about it with others, you begin to attract what's in alignment with that future. This is a very powerful success weapon because it allows you to "visualize your way to reality"—and arrive there.

It's too easy to forget a North Star goal you set a few weeks ago. That's why we like having reminders and cues around us. Examples: set your computer or smartphone wallpaper with the goal on it or stick a small poster on your wall in front of your workspace. The point of the reminder is to set up an environment whereby you *can't* fail.

In Chapter 9, we'll give you specific steps for goal-setting so that you can put together your own plan. What we said under the Believe strategy about attitude, belief, and effort applies to this strategy too. Everything starts with a positive attitude when you want to achieve a goal. When you put your mind to something, then believing in yourself and putting effort into it can take you to astounding heights.

CHAPTER 5

STRATEGY #5: CONNECT

ANYONE WHO HAS BEEN SEXUALLY ABUSED AS A CHILD WILL TELL YOU that it is one of the most isolating and horrific experiences a person can be forced to endure. Yet this heinous act occurs far too often. Sadly, its emotional pain lasts long after the abuse has ended and can have a deeply painful impact on every part of someone's life. Kifa, from our Costa Mesa, California, camp, knows this all too well.

Kifa's childhood was marred by childhood abuse from her biological father and sexual abuse from her stepfather. It was a deeply traumatic experience that left a profound scar on her psyche.

"It bothers you all your life. It shattered my sense of safety, trust, and self-worth," she said. "It decimates you as a human being."

Kifa's mother continued the isolation and trauma by turning a blind eye, not believing what happened was true. This put an extra burden and hardship on Kifa. She became angry, anxious, and depressed. She learned to disassociate. To be silent.

Her mother and others in the family piled on with emotional abuse, making her feel as though it were her fault.

As a teenager, Kifa got pregnant and became a single mom, barely making it with no clear path for the future. She was lost.

But in 2021, she made the life-changing decision to join one of our camps. Immersing herself in the experience, Kifa worked out six days a week, participated in focus meetings with trainers, and connected with other members, which was especially hard for her. Healing from such a profound violation is a long and arduous journey, requiring immense strength and support. She trusted no one; after all, she had once trusted her father, stepfather, and family, only to be betrayed.

But Kifa was not going to let the abuse define the rest of her life. She learned to value herself and her abilities. As she gained strength, she developed so much self-confidence that she enlisted in the US Marines and began rebuilding a life for herself and her son. Kifa is now working toward becoming an officer. She consistently scores at the top of her class with feats that include 90-pound presses, twenty-five strike push-ups, three-minute planks, and weighted hikes. She attributes her success 100 percent to the support she received by connecting to the Burn community. Her physical transformation has been remarkable, but her inner strength and the life she took back are the real heart of her story.

Creating lasting change in your life can be hard on your own. Often, you feel that you're on an island with no one to talk to or support you. It's tough and isolating. Not going to lie to you: without support, you're going to be treading water and getting nowhere fast toward your goals. Connection gives you strength, encouragement, and inspiration to keep going even when you feel as if you can't take another step.

Through our work and interaction with our members, we've found that social connection is one of the most basic aspects of living a healthy and happy life. We're social animals. We depend on other people for survival. We've thrived as a species not because we're swift or strong or have developed weapons, but because of social protection. Our early ancestors, for example, could slay large animals for food only by hunting in groups. Our strength and survival lies in our ability to bond and work together.

In a world where true connections are fading, remember that just as we hunger for food and seek shelter, our soul craves genuine human bonds. The desire to be loved, to fit in at school, to play on a team, to join a club, or to avoid rejection and loss—these things drive a huge array of our thoughts, actions, and feelings.

Over the past fifty years, however, our social connections have been dissolving. We volunteer less. We don't invite guests to our homes much anymore. We're staying single more than ever. We're not having as many kids. We live farther away from our closest relatives. And we have fewer close friends in whom we can confide and find support.

Denying our social nature comes with a price. Over the same period of time that we've become so socially isolated, our degree of happiness has gone down, while rates of suicide and depression have multiplied. Related to this trend is loneliness. At any one moment, nearly one in every two Americans is experiencing measurable levels of loneliness, according to the US surgeon general.

Clearly, social connection is more vital to life than we realize—and it comes with many other benefits. Having strong social bonds is as good for you as healthy behaviors like eating right, exercising, or quitting smoking. Bonding with others also makes you happier—especially when you know they need your help. Connecting even guards against cardiovascular disease, diabetes, mental illness, and other serious conditions.

If you want to rise to another level, you can do it with our Connect strategy.

THE CONNECT STRATEGY HELPS YOU ACHIEVE YOUR NORTH STAR GOALS.

You influence the people around you, for good or bad, and they influence you. It's well known in sociology that behaviors ranging from enjoying a hobby to smoking can spread infectiously through social networks. So can such behaviors as overeating. If your friends are obese, your risk of obesity is 45 percent higher!

In marriages and cohabitation situations, research shows that couples can share bad habits, such as abusing alcohol or gorging on junk food. But what about the opposite? Can good habits rub off too? A study of more than 3,700 cohabiting and married couples, all over the age of fifty, says—yes.

The participants had been given questionnaires every four years since 2002 as a part of an ongoing study on aging that examined the health status and lifestyle among older residents of the UK. The investigators found that men and women shed more weight, got more active, and were more successful at quitting smoking when their partner was pursuing the same health goals.

That's great proof of the power of connection, but we don't always have to turn to science to learn how relationships can improve our lives. We work with a lot of husbands and wives. All it takes is for one of the spouses to get into the act—and boom, the other spouse follows. Here's a story from Gaige at our Highland, Utah, camp.

Embarking on the Burn Boot Camp journey was a transformative experience that I never anticipated. Initially, I hesitated to join, dismissing workout classes as something tailored for women, but my wife, inspired by her own postpartum fitness journey, convinced me to give it a shot. Comfortable in my dad bod but aware of the need for a change, I decided to commit to shedding 30 pounds for the sake of my health and personal aspirations.

The first camp was a wake-up call, pushing me to my limits and leaving me breathless, but it ignited a fire within me. From that point on, I was hooked on the intensity and camaraderie of Burn Boot Camp. Through unwavering consistency, I found that Burn not only helped me surpass my fitness goals but also fostered a sense of belonging within the growing Burn community. Now, as a firm believer, I am not only transforming physically but also embracing the strength and support that comes from being a part of an empowering community.

You're more likely to prioritize exercise when your family, friends, and coworkers are working out too. The daily practice of demanding workouts, the social support, and the camaraderie can spill over into your everyday life, making you a better person, someone who is capable of setting goals and achieving them.

THE CONNECT STRATEGY KEEPS YOU ACCOUNTABLE.

A by-product of community is accountability. So, what does "accountability" mean? Accountability is taking ownership and responsibility for your choices—what you eat, how much you work out, and how you progress toward your North Star goals.

So many are "this close" to breaking through. But there's a problem. They blame other people, things, and circumstances for why they're failing. We get it. But blaming outside circumstances is a losing formula 100 percent of the time.

When you place your expectations for your life and health on yourself instead of a workout program, fad diet, or other people, you win, because it's human nature to meet your own standards. Placing expectations externally on people, things, or events will lead to disappointment because they don't live up to them. Plus, it gives you the opportunity to place blame. Success lies in taking ownership of your actions—there's no one to blame but yourself because you own every decision you make.

If you look a little deeper, you'll realize that it's tougher to hit your goals when you don't feel accountable. Accountability is a huge factor in determining the likelihood of success in all things, from achieving your goals to feeling your best.

You can hold yourself accountable in two ways—by yourself and with others. Ways to hold yourself accountable include tracking your food and workout progress, reviewing pictures of yourself from before you started working out, and remembering what you've done well.

You don't have to do this alone. Find someone you trust as an accountability partner. Check in with them and let them help you stay on course. If you're part of a gym community, you'll be surrounded by positive people who are rooting for your success.

You are accountable for what goes on in your life. When accountability is present, you can keep your eye on a very clear prize.

If we could give one additional piece of advice on accountability, it's not about exercise or diet or habit change. It's about walking your talk and believing in yourself. Because when it's all said and done, it's not a burpee or a salad that produces change. It's accountability to your word—never breaking promises to yourself. At Burn Boot Camp, this is one of our core values. Put another way, we say what we mean, match our actions to our words, and take responsibility for both.

THE CONNECT STRATEGY IS GOOD FOR YOUR HEALTH.

What are friends for? Your good health! You need them. Or else, the opposite of social connection—loneliness—kicks in, often with serious side effects. Loneliness has now been deemed more harmful to your health than obesity, and it's about as deadly as smoking!

Decades of research have linked loneliness to poor health. Case in point: a landmark study conducted in 1979 found that the risk of dying over a nine-year period more than doubled for people with the fewest social connections, compared to those with the most.

Since then, researchers have found even more evidence linking social ties with protection against life-crushing illnesses. For example, strong relationships help protect the heart. In one study, women with heart disease were more than twice as likely to be alive after two years if they were a part of a wide social circle. What's more, they were less likely to develop high blood pressure and diabetes.

Research has also shown that a lack of social connection sparks inflammation and changes in how the immune system works.

In a study published in *Proceedings of the National Academy of Sciences*, researchers from the University of California and University of Chicago discovered that the genes responsible for inflammation were more active in elderly people who were isolated, and genes that help defend against viral infections were depressed. These results suggest that if you're socially isolated, you might be more susceptible to inflammation (which underlies many illnesses) and less able to fight off viral infections.

To prevent these health problems, proactively manage your own social life. Reach out to people, become a hub for physical gatherings of friends, volunteer, or join something! We don't believe you can sit back and wait for someone else to be the leader in this regard. Stop what you're doing, text five people you like and respect, tell them you miss their company and want more, set a date to meet them, and be the leader.

THE CONNECT STRATEGY STRENGTHENS RELATIONSHIPS.

Think about how you feel after a person has truly understood you during a good conversation, or the feeling you get when someone tells you "great job," or the joy of cuddling with someone you love. This is the power of loving, supportive relationships.

It's worth repeating that relationships are at the core of a truly successful life. These include friendships with people you know well, enjoy, and trust. Family is crucial too. And "family" can look like lots of different things.

Have you ever pushed one of your kids on a swing? They might just be sitting there until you give them a push. And you know what happens when you give them a push? Pretty soon, they're pumping and swinging high on their own. That's what our members do in our camps and in gyms everywhere—they give each other a push, and in doing so, everyone grows mutually, feels encouraged, and experiences acceleration and momentum in life.

It's worthwhile here to recall that the pandemic forced many of us into isolation. A lot of people who were missing the gym during that time were not just missing exercise, but being part of something. There's a certain joy and satisfaction in being considered "a regular," no matter where it is. There is always a space made just for you and will be exactly what you need—your only job is to find it!

At camp, we focus on more than just physical transformation. Imagine each of our camps as a firepit, a central gathering place where we come together, not just to work out but to deeply connect and share life's experiences. You don't go to the bonfire for the fire—you go for the connection with your friends. Push-ups are what we do—but it's not *why* we do it.

Some other guidance about building relationships: they are great, but only a good thing if the relationships are good. To maintain good ones, practice forgiveness, communicate honestly, be there for those you love, balance your independence with dependence, and act with care, encouragement, and responsibility toward others. We'll show you how to make this happen in Chapter 10.

THE CONNECT STRATEGY BUILDS INNER STRENGTH.

The opposite of connection is social isolation—and it can threaten our very being. In humans, social isolation is relieved by forming attachments. When an infant cries out in distress, this calls the mother to tend to the baby's needs. In studies of rats and their pups, when mothers did not answer a distress call, the pups often died within two days of birth. Like plants, we grow in the soil of attachment, not isolation, and we need social connection just to exist!

Without connection, you're inviting anxiety and depression into your life. One of our personal experiences really drives this point home. Devan speaking here:

Playing baseball and being part of a team made me feel like I belonged to something—a bunch of individuals all bonded over a common goal that we were motivated to achieve, personally and collectively.

After I was suddenly fired from the team, I was devastated. Then I was angry—beyond angry, in fact. I was furious. I ripped off my Giants' hat and threw it against the door. As powerfully as I could, I stood over the bed and just threw punches on punches on punches at the poor bed. After about thirty minutes of fury, I came up with heavy breath. I picked up my hat and put it back on and walked over to the sink. I put my hands on the sink and leaned into the mirror to stare back at myself for the next five minutes, speechless. As tears welled up in my eyes, I felt a wave of depression for the first time ever. I was lost without my teammates and the common goal of winning. I felt alone. I was a baseball player—that's all I ever wanted to be, all I ever was, and all that worked for me.

Disconnection and rejection are rough on your psyche! But you can overcome such experiences of despair by reconnecting to people and regaining bits and pieces of social interactions. The more we have a sense of inclusion or a sense of being appreciated, or liked or loved, the stronger our inner strength. The group exercise experience, for one thing, can cultivate within us the traits of being compassionate and kind, and loving ourselves.

Our members, for example, tell us that they came for their body but they stayed for their mind. A good example is Elaine, from our Bethel Park, Pennsylvania, camp. Elaine struggled with depression and anxiety all her life, and she never exercised.

She admits to having some very rough days. "I felt like hopelessness had been attached to me for years. It would intensify just when I needed hope the most," she said. "I'd zigzag from optimism to despair and back again. Every day was different, and I muddled my way through."

There are few things more isolating than being depressed, and there is little that can ramp up depression more than being in isolation. Fortunately, a friend asked her to try one of our camps. With the encouragement of her husband, Elaine gave it whirl, although with a lot of hesitation.

"I was so nervous the first day that I forgot my shoes. I borrowed some and I completed my first camp. I fell in love with it fast, and four years later, I'm working out six days a week."

For Elaine, the big draw was the supportive atmosphere. Everyone rallied around her and helped her see that her body was capable of doing so much more than she knew.

"Because of this, I'm the happiest I've ever been. My lifelong battle with depression and anxiety has decreased to basically nonexistent. This place is my therapy. I'm forever grateful."

You have lots of options when it comes to exercise. Always keep in mind that although exercise helps keep you in shape, its greater purpose is for us to live well, feel good, and be productive. When done as a part of the group, these benefits multiply.

OKAY. WHAT'S IT GOING TO TAKE?

We need connection with others now more than ever. We're living in difficult times; we're very separated from others. We're cut off by remote work. We're detached from faith, spirituality, and a Higher Power. We don't connect enough with our body; we don't connect with one another.

You can begin to change all that—now. Here's some groundwork to start laying out.

Take Time for Self-Reflection

Right now might be a good time to evaluate the state of your relationships. Really think about this. Who is in your life now? Who loves you? Who can you call and talk to right now for help and support? Who is an encourager? Who is toxic (it's okay to ditch them!)?

Step back from the chaos of modern life and take the pulse of your relationships. Be honest with yourself about where you're devoting your time and whether you're nurturing the connections that help you thrive. Finding the time for this type of reflection is challenging, and sometimes it's uncomfortable. But it can be incredibly advantageous.

Then make an intentional, sincere commitment to surround yourself with people who inspire, encourage, and motivate you. This is why we created Burn Boot Camp—it's a second home where people can come together to achieve greatness, without one ounce of negativity. We believe that connection is one of the biggest components to happiness and success.

We always say that you'll reflect the five people you hang out with, so a crucial decision in life is figuring out your circle of influence. We'll get to that in Chapter 10, but for now, really give some thought to your relationships and where they stand.

Show Up!

There's a quote on the walls in our gyms: "You showed up, now show up." This message has deep meaning to us. But what should it mean to you?

It's simple, really. It's a daily commitment to prioritize the things that mean the most to your existence as a human being.

Your first job is to show up for yourself. Recognize your worth and take intentional steps to invest in your physical, emotional, and mental health. Take the time, make an effort, commit to your goals and desires, and put yourself first. In other words, you showed up at camp; now, work hard. You're shopping at the grocery store; make good choices. When journaling, be honest about how you feel. Ask yourself the tough questions, do the hard things, and you'll be able to show up for your goals with consistency.

The second is showing up for your cherished relationships with unwavering dedication. Realize the profound impact your presence can have on your family and friends, and vice versa. Be there to connect, make sacrifices when you need to, weather storms with resilience, and celebrate the wins. Together.

The truth is, becoming the person you want to be, surrounded by the people you want to be with, is not rocket science. It simply requires you to show up, for yourself and for them, day after day.

Reach Out

Don't be shy. Reach out to others. If you look at the numbers around loneliness and you realize that there are more people struggling with loneliness than have diabetes in this country—maybe it's a smart move to change your default a little bit in terms of approaching other people. Rather than assuming that people are connected and great and fine, recognize there's a very real chance that the person next to you in an exercise class or elsewhere might be struggling with loneliness. Remind yourself to go the extra mile a little bit, introduce yourself, and ask how they're doing. We have more connection strategies for you in Chapter 10.

There are many forms of connection. You can connect with a workout partner, someone to talk to for encouragement; a professional such as a trainer, counselor, or nutritionist who can provide informational support; a colleague at work; a close family member—anyone who believes in you and wants to see you win. Even social media can offer support! You can even connect directly with us. We spend at least an hour every night engaging with people and their goals. The point is to reach out, show up, empower people, and feel empowered in the process.

PART 2

CREATE THE LIFE YOU LOVE

CHAPTER 6

LET'S GET MOVING

HERE'S THE KIND OF STORY ABOUT WORKING OUT THAT WE LOVE AND hear all the time—this one from Eliza, from Verona, Wisconsin.

Three years ago, Eliza weighed 300 pounds and was in an abusive marriage. On top of everything else, she was addicted to alcohol, food, and cigarettes. Her life was intertwined with miserable habits that brought comfort but also trapped her in a cycle of unhealthiness that had her reeling out of control. After struggling to climb a flight of stairs, her heart racing, and fighting to breathe, she knew she was at the tipping point.

"I didn't feel good about myself, and I was terrified for my future," Eliza said. "I had to turn things around."

She quit drinking, left her husband, began a walking program, and started eating more nutritiously. These efforts paid off, and she noticed small, positive changes in her body. Then she hit a plateau, and her progress stalled.

Eliza felt she needed more intensity with exercise than walking provided. She was nervous about taking the next step with a more physically demanding activity, but she knew she didn't want to go backward. She started attending our Fitchburg, Wisconsin, camp, showing up at five thirty every morning and going through an entire workout most days of the week.

It paid off. Eliza was amazed by her own progress. "I never thought I'd be able to run a mile, do thirty push-ups, or even a single pull-up. I can do all of these things now. I was also able to completely kick my smoking habit and lose 150 pounds."

Eliza added that the encouragement from the community, the way everyone pushes one another, believes in one another, and celebrates one another, was a huge part of her success.

> After I started working out consistently, I noticed not only physical changes but changes to my mindset and how I was feeling. Once you feel happy, you never want to feel unhappy again, and I had forgotten how good it felt to feel good. I started being more conscious about my choices when it came to food, sleep, my relationship with others, and my work.
>
> I got to a healthy place physically, mentally, and emotionally. Most importantly, I now believe in myself, and I have my life back.

Eliza discovered that exercise is the best medicine, and as we've emphasized, working out is extraordinarily therapeutic—physically, mentally, emotionally, and spiritually. Bottom line: less couch time is the first step toward an overall healthier lifestyle and the easiest step to take.

As we said, the CDC defines *sufficient* exercise activity as 150 minutes of moderate activity—that's just two and a half hours—in one week. Or 75 minutes of vigorous activity a week—which is one hour and fifteen minutes.

Do you meet either target?

After we got Burn Boot Camp up and running all over the nation, we attracted people from all ages—men and women who want the strength, energy, and cognitive boost to face the challenges of their personal and professional lives through demanding workouts. We've seen people raise their self-esteem and self-confidence and feel positive and happy in their lives. We've seen people achieve great and attractive bodies they're proud of. Best of all, we've seen them prove to themselves they're capable of accomplishing whatever they want in life.

Say you don't have access to one of our camps. You can connect with us On Demand in our app, but you also have access to all the benefits of our workouts right here. In this chapter, we've got two sets of fourteen workouts for you, covering two levels—Beginner and Advanced.

You've got an opportunity to enter a constant, never-ending cycle of improvement. Why not commit right now?

Don't miss this chance to change your quality of life in all eight areas mentioned in Chapter 4 with one simple belief: "My workouts are the anchor to my life." Transformation starts with one small win, so make the decision to start and never stop!

Need help in getting started?

Begin by coming up with a ritual around your workouts. A ritual is a simple habit you do on a consistent basis without giving it a second thought. There is no effort or practice involved once it's implemented—it's a default action. Rituals create discipline, and discipline is like a muscle. The more you flex and work your discipline muscle, the stronger it gets.

To create a ritual around fitness, ask yourself: "How will I make time for training? What time of day will I work out? How often will I train? What commitment will I make to my training, even when I don't feel like it? Who am I going to train with?"

Say you want to work out first thing in the morning before you go to work every weekday. You might create a ritual in which you get up, eat breakfast, do a workout, shower, get dressed, and head to work. The value of such a ritual is to accustom your mind and body to including exercise in your morning routine (or whatever time of day you like to work out)—so much that you no longer have to think about it; it becomes a second-nature habit for you.

Maybe you do it with a friend, a group of friends, or a trainer—someone who can hold you accountable. Once you get going, you'll find that this simple ritual translates into greater power and more discipline in every area of your life. You'll begin feeling better and happier almost right away.

The way you feel determines how you perform, how you interact with others, and how much you enjoy life—everything! Rigorous, demanding training translates to building an extraordinary life if you'll let it.

THE BURN WORKOUTS YOU CAN DO ANYWHERE

Our gyms use twenty-five-plus pieces of the best fitness equipment made. Our locations offer fourteen different "protocols" (daily workouts) that target different muscle groups and are spaced throughout the week to prevent injury and add variety to your workouts, keeping them interesting and fun. You'll never do the same workout twice. Our app's On Demand feature mirrors our in-gym daily protocol.

For the purposes of this book, we made each protocol bodyweight only in case you don't have access to equipment like weights and bands. You can do these workouts anywhere—at home, in a gym, outdoors, or in a hotel room on vacation. The price is right too. About all you need to spend money on is a pair of good athletic shoes and an exercise mat (although a soft carpeted floor will do nicely too!).

GETTING STARTED

1. Find a suitable space—enough to move around in comfortably without obstructions. Clear the area of any furniture or objects that might get in your way during your workout.

2. Use a soft workout surface. If possible, perform your workouts on a relatively soft surface that provides cushioning and reduces the impact on your joints. Mats, exercise pads, or even carpeted areas are suitable options.

3. Gather together the necessary equipment. Because these workouts use your bodyweight only, you don't need much equipment. However, we do recommend having a stopwatch or timer on hand to keep track of your workout duration and rest periods.

4. Stay hydrated! Keep a filled water bottle nearby. Drink water before, during, and after your workout to replenish fluids lost through sweat.

5. Keep a towel or two handy to wipe away sweat and to use as a cushion or support for certain exercises that may require you to be on your knees or elbows. Additionally, a small towel can help with gripping or reducing friction during certain movements.

6. Read through the exercise descriptions in Appendix A to familiarize yourself with the moves. Then follow proper form and technique, as described in the instructions. It's better to perform the exercises correctly at a slower pace than rush through them with incorrect form. Proper form and technique ensure that you get the maximum results and minimize the risk of injury.

7. Select your fitness level. If you're relatively new to exercising or haven't been consistently active, start with the Beginner workouts. They are designed to introduce you to the exercises, build a foundation of strength and endurance, and help you gradually increase your intensity as you progress. You don't want to jump into the Advanced workouts if you are a beginner, or else you could develop excessive fatigue, soreness, or even injuries.

If you're already familiar with bodyweight exercises and have performed them correctly in the past, you can consider starting with the Advanced workouts. They involve more challenging exercises, higher repetitions, and longer durations. Again, proper form is essential.

8. Evaluate your current strength and endurance levels. If you feel confident in performing exercises that involve multiple muscle groups and you can maintain proper form throughout a variety of moves, you may be ready for the Advanced workouts. On the other hand, if you struggle with basic bodyweight exercises or have limited stamina, we advise that you start with the Beginner workouts so as to gradually build your strength and endurance.

9. Consider the time you can allocate to your workouts. Beginner workouts are generally shorter, making them more suitable if you have time constraints or prefer shorter, high-intensity sessions. The Advanced workouts usually take more time because they're longer and include additional rounds of exercises.

10. Reflect on your fitness goals and what you expect to achieve by following the Burn strategy. If you primarily want to improve your overall fitness, reduce body fat, or increase your strength, the Beginner workouts can provide an excellent starting point. The Advanced workouts may be more appropriate if you have specific goals such as competing in a challenging event, increasing muscular endurance, or achieving other advanced fitness milestones.

11. Focus. With these workouts, you've got to concentrate as if you were commuting to work in busy, snarled traffic. We've seen a lot of people's minds wander while they work out. Learn to feel every exercise. Learn to focus on the muscles you're working. Learn to concentrate on posture, range of motion, position, and repetitions. If you do this, you'll vastly improve!

THE BURN DYNAMIC WARM-UP

This is the initial phase of each workout. It prepares your body for the upcoming exercises and involves a series of moves that increase your heart rate, warm up your muscles, and improve your range of motion. It also activates and engages your major muscle groups, lubricates your joints, and mentally preps you for the workout ahead. Perform each of the dynamic warm-up exercises with controlled, deliberate motions in order to prevent injury and optimize performance.

THE BURN WORKOUTS

The workouts are a combination of bodyweight exercises, conditioning intervals, and strength building. The exercises and format may vary, depending on the routine you perform.

Full-Body Strength

This strength-building routine focuses on the entire body, using your own bodyweight as resistance. We always tell our members, "Don't use machines; be one." All you need is your bodyweight, and you have a gym that travels with you 24/7/365.

This routine:

- Builds body and muscle strength
- Gives you the most workout in the least amount of time
- Burns more calories in a short time
- Protects your health against illnesses
- Helps reserve mental clarity, stimulate neuron growth and activity in the brain, and helps prevent the degenerative effects of aging on the brain
- Enhances mental well-being by releasing mood-lifting chemicals
- Stimulates testosterone and growth hormone production—factors that indirectly improve the formation of muscles and the burning of body fat

Upper-Body Strength

The upper body refers to your arms, forearms, shoulders, back, and chest. Strengthening these areas improves posture, performance, and confidence.

Upper-body strength is super important for your health, and you can test it with a simple exercise, such as the push-up. Proof: in a study published in *JAMA Network Open*, men capable of completing at least forty push-ups in thirty seconds had much lower odds of experiencing a heart attack, heart failure, and other cardiovascular problems than those who could do fewer than ten repetitions in that same time frame.

This routine also:

- Improves coordination
- Develops stronger arms for such sports as swimming, golf, basketball, baseball, and many daily activities, such as putting groceries away
- Decreases injury risks

Lower-Body Strength

With a strong lower body, your everyday functional movements will improve, everything from walking and getting up from your chair to squatting and hiking. You'll not only strengthen your larger muscles but also improve your balance and stamina and decrease the risk of injuries to your knees and hips as well as your risk of falling.

This routine also:

- Tightens and sculpts your glutes, thighs, and hamstrings
- Helps you hit your fitness goals—like running faster or hiking farther

Leg Day

Never skip a leg day! Legs hold you up, and training them should be a top priority. Leg workouts are thus a central feature of a whole-body workout because they build strength, speed, and stability.

This routine also:

- Maximizes and boosts athletic performance for nearly every sport
- Promotes stability in the knee
- Works your heart and lungs. Challenging these larger muscles requires more energy, which means your heart and lungs get a conditioning benefit.
- Improves functional fitness for activities such as picking up boxes, carrying groceries, or moving furniture
- Prevents back pain by strengthening weak hamstrings and short and tight hip flexors
- Tones and sculpts legs
- Burns calories and promotes fat loss (because you're working large muscle groups)

Arm Day

Your arms include a bunch of different muscles, including your biceps (muscles along the front of your upper arms), triceps (the back of your upper arms), deltoids (shoulders), and forearms. Having stronger arms can give you a feeling of confidence. They also convey a sense of athleticism and strength. But there are some important practical benefits to having stronger arms too. Strong arms:

- Promote functional fitness for daily activities, such as pushing a door open or pulling it closed, or simply lifting heavy objects
- Look toned and sculpted
- Assist larger muscles in their moves
- Prevent injuries

Push and Pull

Instead of grouping your training by muscle group or function, push-pull programs alternate between push and pull movements (usually as supersets).

The push moves emphasize pushing actions, which typically involve the chest, shoulders, and triceps. The pull exercises focus on pulling movements, involving the back and biceps.

This routine:

- Promotes muscle size and strength
- Stimulates more muscle fibers and creates a larger release of growth hormone
- Prevents injuries

Full-Body Strength and Conditioning

Conditioning workouts like this are designed to improve strength, power, muscular endurance, and conditioning fitness. Specifically, this workout:

- Builds strength
- Enhances mobility
- Develops core stability
- Enhances heart health
- Reduces the risk of injury
- Improves coordination
- Stabilizes your joints

Burst Training

This unique form of conditioning, burst training, involves short, intense bursts of training lasting 30 to 60 seconds and then 30 to 60 seconds of low-impact or active recovery. It's great for boosting metabolism, managing stress (it reduces and regulates stress hormones), and gives you other benefits as well. For example, burst training:

- Burns fat for nearly 36 hours after your workout
- Improves conditioning fitness
- Enhances overall fitness
- Saves time

Plyometrics

Plyometrics, often called jump training, is a type of exercise that uses the speed and force of distinct movements to build muscle power. It boosts metabolism and improves sports performance.

Plyometric training also:

- Builds muscular power (ability to apply force quickly)
- Prevents athletic injuries
- Enhances an athlete's vertical jump (ability to make quick lateral movements), punching/kicking force, and running speed

Speed and Agility

Speed is the ability to move quickly and relies on muscular strength and endurance. Agility, on the other hand, is the ability to move quickly in one direction and then instantly decelerate and shift your position within seconds. Training for speed and agility:

- Gives athletes an extra-competitive edge
- Improves balance and coordination to help athletes be more stable and nimble on their feet
- Helps strengthen those muscles that usually fatigue easily during competition
- Helps you push yourself harder without increasing your risk of injury

Core Strength and Conditioning

Core training focuses on improving power, posture, agility, and stability. **A strong core is the foundation of the entire body and is a staple to the program.** Core training:

- Prevents injury
- Builds back strength
- Prevents lower back pain
- Increases the endurance performance of your core muscles
- Improves balance
- Strengthens performance in such sports as golf and tennis

Bodyweight Conditioning

This routine targets your entire body, activating various muscle groups to condition your body and develop cardiovascular endurance. The workout combines several types of exercises, from conditioning to resistance training using your own bodyweight.

Body conditioning:

- Boosts endurance
- Enhances joint flexibility
- Improves mobility for daily activities
- Creates a balanced, stable physique
- Promotes better functional movement

Athletic Conditioning

With a combination of strength training and serious conditioning work, this workout is designed to improve sport performance. You'll become a better all-around athlete, even improve as a "weekend warrior," whether that's for softball, basketball, tennis, golf, bicycling, skiing, hiking, or paddle sports. This workout also:

- Helps boost your brainpower, since practicing athletic drills helps you increase your motor skills and works your cognitive skills
- Enhances reaction time
- Boosts your coordination and overall performance in fitness

Metabolic Conditioning

Designed to reset and boost metabolism, this routine uses very specific and timed groups of exercises that strengthen your whole body; improve your speed, agility, balance, and coordination; and build conditioning. This workout also:

- Boosts your metabolism for many hours after you work out
- Primes your metabolism to work faster to burn more fat
- Pushes your body to help you develop lean muscle mass

The primary goal of all these workouts is to challenge and push your body, improve endurance, build strength, and most importantly, gain confidence. You'll employ a variety of exercises, including squats, lunges, push-ups, planks, burpees, mountain climbers, and more.

Some workouts incorporate "intervals." These are periods of intense effort punctuated by short periods of rest or active recovery to maintain the intensity and maximize your results.

These workouts conclude with a "finisher." Performed at the end, these include a short but intense series designed to provide a final burst of effort and leave you feeling accomplished. Finishers push your limits and challenge your endurance. By performing finishers, you increase the intensity of your workout, stimulate muscle growth, and activate the afterburn effect. The afterburn effect, also known as excess postexercise oxygen consumption (EPOC), refers basically to the increased quantity of calories burned after exercise is complete.

REPS AND ROUNDS

This might sound a little elementary, but just so we're on the same page, we want to explain that you'll do each exercise a certain number of times. Each time you do a single move, it's called a "rep," shorthand for "repetition." So, if a workout says "10 reps," you perform that move ten times. A number of reps done together is a "set." Also, note that "2:1" means doing both sides once = 1 rep.

A key point about reps is control. If you lose control of the rep, you're doing it too fast. If you do it too fast, you're not getting the full benefit of the move. You want to feel the muscle working.

Exercises are grouped into "rounds." This is a sequence of two or more exercises performed in order, one right after the other. In most cases, you'll do a round, then repeat it multiple times.

Several of the workouts employ "supersets." With a superset, you perform two exercises back-to-back with no rest period in between. This training technique increases the intensity (effort) in a workout, helps develop more strength and lean muscle, burns more calories, and is great for fitness.

Okay, let's get to it!

BEGINNER-LEVEL WORKOUTS

(Exercise instructions are found in Appendix A.)

Full-Body Strength

+ **The Dynamic Warm-Up**

Perform the warm-up for a sequence of two rounds.

Jumping Jacks—20 seconds

Shoulder Taps—20 seconds

Squats—20 seconds

+ **The Workout**

Perform the workout for a sequence of two rounds. After
each round, rest for 20 seconds.

Push-Ups—40 seconds

Glute Bridges—40 seconds

Plank-Ups—40 seconds

Calf Raises—40 seconds

+ **The Finisher**

Perform one round.

Low Plank Hold—90 seconds

Upper-Body Strength

+ **The Dynamic Warm-Up (3 minutes)**

Walkouts—5 reps

Supermans—5 reps

+ **The Workout (4 minutes)**

Push-Ups—10 reps

Chair Tricep Dips—10 reps

Plank-Ups—10 reps

Superman Lat Squeezes—10 reps

+ **The Finisher (1 minute)**

Perform one round.

Diamond Push-Ups for the maximum number of reps you
can do.

Lower-Body Strength

+ The Dynamic Warm-Up

Perform the warm-up for a sequence of three rounds total.

Hamstring Scoops—30 seconds

Low Runner Lunges—30 seconds

+ The Workout

Perform the warm-up for a sequence of three rounds total.
   After each round, rest for 20 seconds.

Reverse Lunges—30 seconds on each leg

Single Leg Glute Bridges—30 seconds on each leg

Wall Sit—60 seconds

+ The Finisher

Perform one round.

Jump Squats—90 seconds

Leg Day

+ The Dynamic Warm-Up (3 minutes)

Butt Kickers—10 reps (2:1 [2 sides = 1 rep])

Squats—10 reps

+ The Workout

Perform the following two exercises back-to-back (this is
   referred to as a "superset") for a total of two rounds. Rest
   for 20 seconds between supersets.

Sumo Squats—10 reps

Chair Step-Ups—10 reps each leg

Forward Lunges—15 reps each leg

Perform the following superset for a total of two rounds.
   Rest for 20 seconds between supersets

Glute Bridges—20 reps

Calf Raises—20 reps

+ The Finisher

Perform one round.

Split Squats—25 reps per leg

Arm Day

+ **The Dynamic Warm-Up**

Perform the warm-up for a sequence of two rounds total.

Rapid Fire Punches—40 seconds

Shoulder Taps—40 seconds

+ **The Workout**

Perform the workout sequence for four rounds total. After each round, rest for 20 seconds.

Chair Tricep Dips—40 seconds

Plank-Ups—40 seconds

Diamond Push-Ups—40 seconds

+ **The Finisher**

Perform one round.

Full Burpees—2 minutes

Push and Pull

+ **The Dynamic Warm-Up (3.5 minutes)**

Arm Circles—10 reps in each direction

Thoracic Rotations—10 reps with each arm

+ **The Workout (14 minutes)**

Renegade Rows—10 reps (2:1)

Superman Lat Squeezes—10 reps

Push-Ups—10 reps

+ **The Finisher**

Shoulder Taps—50 reps (2:1)

Full-Body Strength and Conditioning

+ **The Dynamic Warm-Up**

Perform the warm-up for a sequence of three rounds total.

Jumping Jacks—40 seconds

Mountain Climbers—40 seconds

+ The Workout

Perform the workout for a sequence of three rounds total. After each round, rest for 20 seconds.

Squats—40 seconds

Half Burpees—40 seconds

Low Plank Hold—40 seconds

Alternating Lateral Lunges—40 seconds

+ The Finisher

Perform one round.

Push-Ups—60 seconds

Burst Training

+ The Dynamic Warm-Up

Perform the warm-up for a sequence of three rounds total.

Butt Kickers—20 seconds

Walkouts—20 seconds

+ The Workout

Perform the workout for a sequence of four rounds total. After each round, rest for 10 seconds.

Jump Squats—20 seconds

Full Burpees—20 seconds

Mountain Climbers—20 seconds

+ The Finisher

Perform one round.

Half Burpees—60 seconds

Plyometrics

+ The Dynamic Warm-Up (3.5 minutes)

Low Runner Lunges—5 reps (2:1)

Squats—10 reps

+ The Workout (14 minutes)

Skater Hops—10 reps (2:1)

Jump Squats—20 reps

Heismans—30 reps (2:1)

+ **The Finisher**

Perform one round.

Jump Lunges—30 reps (2:1)

Speed and Agility

+ **The Dynamic Warm-Up**

Perform the warm-up for a sequence of three rounds total.

Mountain Climbers—30 seconds

High Knee Sprinters—30 seconds

+ **The Workout**

Perform the workout for a sequence of three rounds total.

After each round, rest for 10 seconds.

Rapid Fire Punches—30 seconds

Dot Drill—30 seconds

Power Planks—30 seconds

Heismans—30 seconds

+ **The Finisher**

Perform one round.

Skater Hops—75 seconds

Core Strength and Conditioning

+ **The Dynamic Warm-Up (3 minutes)**

Walkouts—5 reps

Scissor Kicks—10 reps (2:1)

+ **The Workout**

Perform the following two exercises back-to-back as a super-
set for two rounds. Rest for 20 seconds between supersets.

Mountain Climbers—20 reps (2:1)

Reverse Crunches—20 reps

Perform the following two exercises back-to-back as a superset for
two rounds. Rest for 20 seconds between supersets.

Half Burpees—20 reps

Bicycle Crunch—20 reps (2:1)

+ The Finisher

Perform one round.

Flutter Kicks—100 reps (2:1)

Bodyweight Conditioning

+ The Dynamic Warm-Up (3.5 minutes)

Hamstring Scoops—8 reps (2:1)

Jumping Jacks—8 reps

+ The Workout (14 minutes)

Full Burpees—8 reps

Push-Ups—8 reps

Jump Squats—8 reps

+ The Finisher

Perform one round.

Low Side Plank Hold—45-second hold per side

Athletic Conditioning

+ The Dynamic Warm-Up

Perform the warm-up sequence for three rounds.

Rapid Fire Punches—30 seconds

Butt Kickers—30 seconds

+ The Workout

Perform the workout for a sequence of three
  rounds total. After each round, rest for
  10 seconds.

Bear Crawls—60 seconds

Half Burpees—60 seconds

Heismans—60 seconds

+ The Finisher

Perform one round.

Wall Sit—2 minutes

Metabolic Conditioning

+ The Dynamic Warm-Up (3.5 minutes)

Low Runner Lunges—5 reps (2:1)

Half Burpees—5 reps

+ The Workout (10 minutes)

Full Burpees—10 reps

Jump Lunges—10 reps (2:1)

Plank-Ups—10 reps (2:1)

+ The Finisher

Perform one round.

Jump Squats—50 reps

ADVANCED-LEVEL WORKOUTS

Full-Body Strength

+ The Dynamic Warm-Up

Perform the warm-up for a sequence of three
    rounds total.

Jumping Jacks—20 seconds

Shoulder Taps—20 seconds

Squats—20 seconds

+ The Workout

Perform the workout for a sequence of five
    rounds total. After each round, rest for
    10 seconds.

Push-Ups—40 seconds

Glute Bridges—40 seconds

Plank-Ups—40 seconds

Calf Raises—40 seconds

+ The Finisher

Perform one round.

Low Plank Hold—2 minutes

Upper-Body Strength

+ **The Dynamic Warm-Up (5 minutes)**

Walkouts—5 reps

Supermans—5 reps

+ **The Workout (28 minutes)**

Push-Ups—10 reps

Chair Tricep Dips—10 reps

Plank-Ups—10 reps

Superman Lat Squeezes—10 reps

+ **The Finisher (90 seconds)**

Perform one round.

Diamond Push-Ups for maximum reps

Lower-Body Strength

+ **The Dynamic Warm-Up**

Perform the warm-up for a sequence of four rounds total.

Hamstring Scoops—30 seconds

Low Runner Lunges—30 seconds

+ **The Workout**

Perform the workout for a sequence of five rounds total.

After each round, rest for 10 seconds.

Reverse Lunges—30 seconds each leg

Single Leg Glute Bridges—30 seconds each leg

Wall Sit—60 seconds

+ **The Finisher**

Perform one round.

Jump Squats—2 minutes

Leg Day

+ **The Dynamic Warm-Up (5 minutes)**

Butt Kickers—10 reps (2:1)

Squats—10 reps

+ The Workout

Perform the following two exercises back-to-back as a super-
set for four rounds. Rest for 20 seconds between supersets.

Sumo Squats—10 reps

Chair Step-Ups—10 reps per leg

Forward Lunges—15 reps each leg

Perform the following two exercises back-to-back as a superset for
four rounds. Rest for 20 seconds between supersets.

Glute Bridges—20 reps

Calf Raises—20 reps

+ The Finisher

Perform one round.

Split Squats—60 reps on each leg

Arm Day

+ The Dynamic Warm-Up

Perform the warm-up for a sequence of three rounds total.

Rapid Fire Punches—40 seconds

Shoulder Taps—40 seconds

+ The Workout

Perform the workout for a sequence of five rounds total.
After each round, rest for 10 seconds.

Chair Tricep Dips—40 seconds

Plank-Ups—40 seconds

Diamond Push-Ups—40 seconds

+ The Finisher

Perform one round.

Full Burpees—2 minutes

Push and Pull

+ The Dynamic Warm-Up (5 minutes)

Arm Circles—10 reps in each direction

Thoracic Rotations—10 reps each arm

+ The Workout (28 minutes)

Renegade Rows—10 reps (2:1)

Superman Lat Squeezes—10 reps

Push-Ups—10 reps

+ The Finisher

Perform one round.

Shoulder Taps—100 reps (2:1)

Full-Body Strength and Conditioning

+ The Dynamic Warm-Up

Perform the warm-up for a sequence of four rounds total.

Jumping Jacks—40 seconds

Mountain Climbers—40 seconds

+ The Workout

Perform the workout for a sequence of five rounds total.

　After each round, rest for 20 seconds.

Squats—40 seconds

Half Burpees—40 seconds

Low Plank Hold—40 seconds

Alternating Lateral Lunges—40 seconds

+ The Finisher

Perform one round.

Push-Ups—75 seconds

Burst Training

+ The Dynamic Warm-Up

Perform the warm-up for a sequence of four rounds total.

Butt Kickers—20 seconds

Walkouts—20 seconds

+ The Workout

Perform the workout for a sequence of six rounds total.

　After each round, rest for 20 seconds.

Jump Squats—20 seconds

Full Burpees—20 seconds
Mountain Climbers—20 seconds
+ **The Finisher**
Perform one round.
Half Burpees—75 seconds

Plyometrics

+ **The Dynamic Warm-Up (5 minutes)**
Low Runner Lunges—5 reps each side (2:1)
Squats—10 reps
+ **The Workout (28 minutes)**
Skater Hops—10 reps (2:1)
Jump Squats—20 reps
Heismans—30 reps (2:1)
+ **The Finisher**
Perform one round.
Jump Lunges—40 reps (2:1)

Speed and Agility

+ **Dynamic Warm-Up**
Perform the warm-up for a sequence of four rounds total.
Mountain Climbers—30 seconds
High Knee Sprinters—30 seconds
+ **The Workout**
Perform the workout for a sequence of six rounds total.
After each round, rest for 20 seconds.
Rapid Fire Punches—30 seconds
Dot Drill—30 seconds
Power Planks—30 seconds
Heismans—30 seconds
+ **The Finisher**
Perform one round.
Skater Hops—90 seconds

Core Conditioning

+ The Dynamic Warm-Up (5 minutes)

Walkouts—5 reps

Scissor Kicks—10 reps (2:1)

+ The Workout

Perform the following two exercises back-to-back as a super-
set. Do four rounds with a 20-second rest period between
each round.

Glute Bridges—20 reps

Calf Raises—20 reps

Perform the following two exercises back-to-back as a superset. Do
four rounds with a 20-second rest period between each round.

Mountain Climbers—20 reps (2:1)

Reverse Crunches—20 reps

Perform the following two exercises back-to-back as a superset. Do
four rounds with a 20-second rest period between each round.

Half Burpees—20 reps

Bicycle Crunch—20 reps

+ The Finisher

Perform one round.

Flutter Kick—200 reps (2:1)

Bodyweight Conditioning

+ The Dynamic Warm-Up (5 minutes)

Hamstring Scoops—8 reps (2:1)

Jumping Jacks—8 reps

+ The Workout (28 minutes)

Full Burpees—8 reps

Push-Ups—8 reps

Jump Squats—8 reps

+ The Finisher

Perform one round.

Low Side Plank Hold—45 seconds hold on each side

Athletic Conditioning

+ The Dynamic Warm-Up

Perform four rounds.

Rapid Fire Punches—30 seconds

Butt Kickers—30 seconds

+ The Workout

Perform the workout for a sequence of six rounds total.

After each round, rest for 20 seconds.

Bear Crawls—60 seconds

Half Burpees—60 seconds

Heismans—60 seconds

+ The Finisher

Perform one round.

Wall Sit—2.5 minutes

Metabolic Conditioning

+ The Dynamic Warm-Up (5 minutes)

Low Runner Lunges—5 reps each side (2:1)

Half Burpees—5 reps

+ The Workout (28 minutes)

Full Burpees—10 reps

Jump Lunges—10 reps (2:1)

Plank-Ups—10 reps (2:1)

+ The Finisher

Perform one round.

Jump Squats—75 reps

PUT IT ALL TOGETHER: ORGANIZE YOUR WEEKLY WORKOUTS.

After you've read over the workouts and the exercise instructions in Appendix A, you'll want to create a weekly routine for yourself. Depending on your performance goals, you may want to focus on certain types of routines, such as strength or conditioning or both. Select the routines that fit your goals and preferences, then organize your week around them. With fourteen workouts from which to choose, you have a lot of variety, and you'll never get bored. Plus, you can change your routines—say, every six weeks—to make sure your body doesn't plateau (when you feel like you want to make further progress or you'd just like to change things up a bit).

Here are three examples of weekly workouts. They illustrate how you can build your week around different workouts. Feel free to use any of these, or create your own weekly routine.

If you've just started exercising or haven't worked out in a while, use the Beginner workouts. Once you are fully into the workouts, you'll want to move up to the Advanced routines.

+ **Sample Week #1 (overall strength and conditioning)**
  Monday—Athletic Conditioning
  Tuesday—Upper-Body Strength
  Wednesday—Metabolic Conditioning
  Thursday—Lower-Body Strength
  Friday—Bodyweight Conditioning
  Saturday—Full-Body Strength
  Sunday—Rest
+ **Sample Week #2 (4 strength, 2 conditioning)**
  Monday—Arm Day
  Tuesday—Plyometrics
  Wednesday—Leg Day
  Thursday—Push and Pull
  Friday—Speed and Agility
  Saturday—Full-Body Strength
  Sunday—Rest
+ **Sample Week #3 (4 conditioning, 2 strength)**
  Monday—Upper-Body Strength
  Tuesday—Athletic Conditioning
  Wednesday—Core Strength and Conditioning

Thursday—Lower-Body Strength
Friday—Bodyweight Conditioning
Saturday—Metabolic Conditioning
Sunday—Rest

One way to build connections and accountability and enjoy yourself is to work out with a partner. A partner can help you stay consistent, push you, and inspire you to stay the course. Inspiration, however, must come from within. We know you have that determination! It makes the difference between the impossible and the possible.

That said, select your partner wisely, because not everyone will make the best partner in the workout department. For example, you should gravitate toward a workout partner who is reliable—someone you can count on, rain or shine; who is knowledgeable and knows what they're doing; and who is positive, with an enthusiastic, encouraging mindset.

Now, with the Burn strategy and Burn workouts, there is only one thing left to do—stick with it. You now have the right workouts to claim all the benefits of a physically active life.

We want you to get excited about working out, and we're excited for you. Not just for the physical results, but also for the psychological benefits of the sheer act of moving your body, the gratitude for being able to do so, and the fun of doing it. Trust us, these workouts will unleash the potential inside you and leave you feeling stronger and more confident in all aspects of your life. They will make you a better, higher-performing person, and help you overcome fear, release anger, exert yourself, and test your character.

CHAPTER 7

WHAT YOU THINK, YOU CREATE

GIVEN A 15 PERCENT CHANCE OF SURVIVAL AFTER BEING DIAGNOSED with a form of leukemia, Tiffany, from our Battle Creek, Michigan, camp, found help and hope in unlikely corners of her life, including physical movement and a renewed belief in herself. Hers is a portrait of resilience. This is her story.

Tiffany's life skidded to an abrupt halt in 2022. She was diagnosed with acute myeloid leukemia, a blood cancer that infiltrates essential components of the body's immune system, creating an excess of white blood cells in the bone marrow.

Before this harrowing diagnosis derailed her life, Tiffany had always been very health conscious. She exercised regularly. She ate a consistently nutritious diet. She had boundless energy.

But as the leukemia began to take over her body, her white blood cell count rose so high that she was rushed to the hospital, without being able to hug or say goodbye to her children.

Most people would ask, "Why me?" but Tiffany ultimately realized that this question was not the right one to ask. The right question was: "What do I need to do to beat this?"

"I started my fight for my children, my husband, and myself, and would keep on fighting until I was home and healthy again. I decided to not let my faith waver nor my will to fight. I thought about all the milestones I would miss if I did not win this battle: graduations, weddings, and grandchildren. The idea of not being there was the saddest of all."

No sooner was Tiffany diagnosed than she was told treatment would begin more or less immediately. The standard medical protocol for this disease is chemotherapy. It involved a rigorous schedule of treatment in the hospital, and it consumed her days. But this particular form of chemo did not work. The doctors had to prepare her for the next step—a stem cell transplant.

Along the way came another blow. Her doctors needed to remove a prediagnosed patch of skin cancer from her nose. A biopsy revealed that the skin cancer was larger than previously thought. Her entire nose had to be removed, and skin from her forehead and scalp was used to rebuild it.

"Not only was I fighting this horrific leukemia, but I now had more than 200 stitches in my face. I knew I would never look the same as I did before, but I refused to feel sorry for myself. I remained positive and moved forward."

During this ordeal, Tiffany's white blood cell count skyrocketed. Another type of chemo was required over time, the goal of which was to kill remaining cancer cells and bring the disease into remission so that she could have the stem cell transplant.

That round of chemo brought complications—an infected picc line (for the infusion of chemo into her body) and a resulting staph infection. Tiffany had a violent allergic reaction to the medicine used to treat the infection.

Her husband visited her in the hospital one day and prayed over her while she was shaking from an extreme fever. After some time in prayer, he heard a message from God: "Get up! Get up! Move!"

"At first, I was too weak to get up or move on my own. I could barely walk unassisted, but my husband helped me. I had lost motor skills and strength. Still, I kept on moving. Then I kept getting better, so I kept moving more. I finally was released from the hospital and, thankfully, had achieved remission and was now a candidate for the transplant. I was told the neurological damage from the last type of chemo could be permanent. I refused to accept that. Devan Kline told me once that a lot of our physical health is linked to our mindset. I fully believed that!"

At home, Tiffany started walking on her treadmill for 2 miles a day at a slow pace. She tightly grasped the rails when her legs wanted to give out. She worked her way up to 5 miles a day. After one week of pushing herself, she could walk normally. A few weeks later, she was riding her mountain bike on the dirt trails by her home.

"I refused to be taken out by this cancer, and I never wavered."

Tiffany checked into the hospital again for further treatment, including the stem cell transplant. The hospital let her bring an exercise bicycle into her room. Although weak and sick from the treatment, she rode the bike for forty-five minutes a day, sometimes twice a day. "Get up and move" became her anthem.

Tiffany was released from the hospital a week earlier than estimated. She returned home, determined and more positive than ever to make the most out of her second chance at life.

"I went back to Burn in October 2022. I made camp five to six days a week, and I would not stop."

Over the course of her journey, Tiffany and her husband spoke to several cancer survivors. All those who beat the odds had one thing in common, but it wasn't just the hospital, the doctors, or the treatments. It was the positive mindset—the same mindset Tiffany maintained from day one.

Today, she says: "I went on an oral chemo drug to prevent the leukemia from returning. I receive frequent blood draws to track my counts. I've had multiple surgeries and procedures on my face. I've hit bumps in the road and setbacks. Regardless of any of this, I don't let the trials get to me. I focus on my victories. I stay positive, and I will never stop fighting."

Tiffany faced each diagnosis with unwavering courage and a fierce determination to live. Her story reminds us all that even in the face of unimaginable adversity, the human capacity for resilience and hope can light the way through the darkest of times.

For Tiffany, the diagnosis was a massive shock, and the news kept getting worse. At times, she couldn't think straight. But she had to become a channel of self-love, get rid of negative emotions, and keep moving forward. Her resilience, emotional strength, attitude, and effort kept her going, thriving, and surviving. The workouts she did—in the hospital, at home, in the gym, outdoors, no matter where—laid a physiological foundation that boosted her mental health and helped her tell her body and spirit that she wanted to live. Most people don't realize the power of their mind—but Tiffany did, and she used it.

Wouldn't you like to develop and strengthen your own focus as Tiffany did? You can, and there are several actions here that you can take to do so. In fact, if you implement just one, you can drastically change your life. Look over our Believe strategy and the exercises it involves. Then determine which ones will serve you best. Focus on the things you need to focus on, because they can alter the course of your life forever.

MASTER EMOTIONAL INTELLIGENCE.

Emotional intelligence is a necessary skill for navigating life. When you're aware of your emotions and express them in a healthy way, professional and personal success is yours.

So, how do you develop it? With one simple step, you can.

Follow a very straightforward process Devan learned during his baseball days. It's called "play back the tape." We're talking about the mental tapes that run through your mind all day long. They contain messages, self-talk, or beliefs that we repeat back to ourselves—and believe. Some tapes are positive messages, while others are negative.

To do this exercise, know that there is always a "shadow" version of you following you all the time. Pretend this version of you is sitting in the corner of every room.

Say you had an interaction, meeting, experience, or event, and it left you with strong emotions, such as anger, frustration, or sadness. Ask your shadow three questions, which will rewind and play the tape in your head:

- What response did I give that was positive and perhaps I'm grateful for it? (I remained calm . . . I understood the opposing position . . . I watched my words.)
- What response did I give that I was not proud of? (I lashed out and lost my temper . . . I was critical . . . I complained.)
- What will I change next time? (I'll be more empathetic and imagine myself in others' positions so that I know how I might feel in their shoes . . . I'll practice active listening to understand someone better . . . I'll look for the positive lesson in the interaction and be grateful . . . I'll stay calm under pressure and focus on finding a solution that helps everyone meet their goals.)

If you do this exercise frequently, you'll develop all the mental muscles it takes to build the qualities of an emotionally intelligent person: self-awareness, emotional regulation, empathy, conflict resolution, resilience, and gratitude.

USE TRANSFORMATIVE LANGUAGE.

For real and lasting transformation, you want your inner commentary—your self-talk—to be positive so that it supports the life change you desire. We dipped our toes in the pool of self-talk in Chapter 2. Now, it's time to go a little deeper.

Begin to "tune in" to your self-talk and be aware of anything that is negative. Awareness is the first step toward transformation.

A simple exercise from our lives:

Our kids have "sight words" given to them by their teachers. These words help them recognize common words faster.

We teach an adult version of sight words. This exercise lets you easily recognize when you're being negative or using disempowering language. Watch for these sight words in how you think, believe, and speak:

Can't	Worse
Won't	Bad
Don't	Terrible
Never	Awful
Always (in negative context, such as "You always do that")	Disgusting
	Hate
	Stupid
No	Ugly
Not	Dirty
Nothing	Horrible
None	Loser
Nobody	Disappointing
Nowhere	Ruin
Neither	Mess
Nor	Disaster
Except	Screw up
But	Let down
Unfortunately	Ridiculous
Impossible	Unfair
Problem	Disagree
Issues	Refuse
Difficult	Deny
Failure	Reject
Wrong	Blame
Mistake	Complain
Regret	Criticize

How many of these words crop up in your self-talk and vocabulary? How often?

If you use any of these words, they are bumps and trip hazards on your path to transformation. To eliminate the disempowering chatter, make a list of the words from the above list that you use most often.

Next, make a habit of replacing them with positive sight words—a process that rewires your brain for positivity. Using the same list:

Can't—Can

Won't—Will

Don't—Do

Never—Always
  (in a positive context)

Always—Seldom
  or rarely

No—Yes

Not—Definitely

Nothing—Everything

None—All

Nobody—Everyone

Nowhere—Everywhere

Neither—Every

Nor—Or, and, or also

Except—Include

But—And, furthermore

Unfortunately—Fortunately

Impossible—Possible

Problem—Challenge

Issues—Unimportant

Difficult—Doable or easy

Failure—Success,
  experience, challenge

Wrong—Right

Mistake—Accurateness,
  learning opportunity

Regret—Be content, accept,
  satisfied

Worse—Matchless, unequalled

Bad—Good

Terrible—Great, excellent, fine

Awful—Awesome, terrific

Disgusting—Agreeable, beautiful,
  decent

Hate—Love

Stupid—Smart

Ugly—Beautiful

Dirty—Clean

Horrible—Delightful, pleasant,
  appealing, enjoyable

Loser—Winner

Disappointing—Satisfying,
  encouraging, rewarding

Ruin—Enrich

Mess—Order, organized

Disaster—Success, godsend

Screw up—Accuracy,
  correctness

Let down—Fulfillment,
  satisfaction, victory

Ridiculous—Reasonable, logical

Unfair—Fair

Disagree—Agree

Refuse—Accept   Blame—Be accountable
Deny—Support   Complain—Compliment
Reject—Accept   Criticize—Encourage

We also recommend that you analyze your day. In a journal or on a piece of paper, create three columns:

- Keep
- Delete
- Upgrade

At the end of the day, play back your mental tapes with the goal of using better self-talk. Under "Keep," record what you loved about your attitude, beliefs, and reactions to events. For instance: I exercised self-control over my behavior. I did "hard things." I handled that situation with calm and confidence.

Under "Delete," write down the things you didn't like that made you feel uneasy. Examples: I can't do it. I'll fail. I'm uncoordinated. I'm too busy.

Under "Upgrade," write down more positive ways you could have reacted or processed those negative thoughts: I can do that. I will be successful. I will make time in my schedule.

Then do your best to make these adjustments—*keep, delete,* or *upgrade.* Be patient with yourself. Attitude change doesn't happen overnight, but over time.

This "Keep/Delete/Upgrade" piece is the framework in which your shadow self can give you feedback.

Gradually, your attitude will change because you'll begin acting in a manner consistent with the mental state you desire. With a healthy positive attitude, you take challenging situations in stride, you learn from experience, and you prepare for success in your next encounter or experience.

You'll then notice that your effort in accomplishing what you want strengthens. Effort is one of the main things that matters when it comes to success. If your attitude is "I'm good at this," you'll put in a powerful effort at it.

You'll also discover that you've become a more positive person. A positive person is an emotionally intelligent person—someone who understands the power of a positive word, an encouraging email, and a kind gesture.

Winners are winners because they've learned to talk like winners. When they talk like winners, they act like winners. When they act like winners, they *are* winners.

CHANGE YOUR SELF-LIMITING BELIEFS.

Have you ever decided not to apply for that better job because you believe you're not qualified enough? Or stayed away from the gym because you believe you're too out of shape or uncoordinated? Or avoided asking a friend for help because you feel that you'd be a nuisance? Sure, we all have. Such beliefs are common, but they hold you back more than you realize, because they are self-limiting.

Self-limiting beliefs are brakes that stop you from achieving your potential. They can keep you from trying new things, taking risks, and reaching for your dreams. They can also lead to feelings of anxiety, depression, and low self-esteem.

Take a look at this list. How many of these self-limiting beliefs do you hold?

- I'll never be fit. Poor health runs in my family.
- I'll never be successful.
- I'm not smart enough.
- I don't earn enough money.
- I'm not talented enough.

- I'm not capable of change.

If you have self-limiting beliefs, it's important to recognize them, and challenge them. Ask yourself:

- Are my beliefs really true? Are they even rational?
- Are they based on facts, or are they just my fears talking?
- Is this what I believe or is it what someone else told me and I believed it all my life?

Once you've questioned your beliefs, you can overcome the negative ones. Start by thinking the opposite. For example, if you think you don't make enough money, start believing that you can earn more money by upgrading your skills, going back to school, or even looking for a better job. Then act on this. Change your thoughts and your beliefs—and you change your life.

At the same time, begin replacing self-limiting beliefs with more positive and empowering beliefs. In the first example, a new empowering belief would be: "I know other people who have changed their lives through fitness. It must be possible. This belief was my past reality, but my new reality is that I can do this."

Believe that you're a person who can do anything you set your mind to, and you'll naturally take actions that bring you extraordinary success.

FOCUS ON OPPORTUNITIES.

Can a single thought turn into reality?

Yes. In Chapter 2, we introduced you to the reticular activating system (RAS), the part of your brain that controls your *attention and alertness* and helps make goals happen. When you're very focused on what you want, you begin to attract people, places, things, and opportunities into your life.

Some examples:

- You've decided to eat nutritiously so you can become healthier and more energetic. You start scrolling through Facebook and your RAS unconsciously spots a relevant and healthy recipe that works with your eating plan. Had you tried to do that consciously, you may not have found it so easily.
- You've been sporadic with your workouts and know you need to get more active and do so with consistency. You're sitting around one day, and all of a sudden, your gym sends you an email with a special on personal training sessions. Suddenly, it's clear that working with a personal trainer is a great solution and the opportunity to do so has just landed in your lap.
- You're out with friends or at a party, and someone brings up the fact that there's a new position open at a successful company—the kind of job you've always wanted and have been focusing on to attain. You've been alerted to it. The power of your RAS just kicked in. It is your great invisible weapon.

The RAS is scanning the horizon of your opportunities all the time. They are all around us, waiting to be grabbed. Take control of that power and make some positive changes.

Okay, let's get to the good stuff. We're going to show you how to use the RAS to your advantage:

- **Establish your North Star goals.** The RAS works hand in hand with those goals. We show you how to set them in Chapter 9. One of the keys to goal-setting, remember, is to write them down—but do this in your own handwriting. The RAS interacts more effectively with handwritten goals than with those typed into your computer, tablet, or smartphone.
- **Align with your beliefs.** Your beliefs about yourself and the world often dictate your actions below your level of awareness.

For example, if you say you'd like to reduce bodyweight and get healthier, but deep down, you don't believe you can do that, then you'll act in ways that subtly support your belief, and it will be challenging to achieve that goal. Keep challenging your beliefs and eliminate those that limit you.

- **Focus, focus, focus.** Think about your goals and the opportunities you want—consistently and with repetition. When you're thinking about these things, you're focusing. Your RAS will act on this and alert you to new opportunities.

It's easy to spot opportunities when you're always focused on opportunities. You become, and achieve, what you constantly focus on.

IDENTIFY YOUR UNIVERSAL NEEDS.

Universal needs are required for us to thrive, flourish, and ultimately live our best lives. Primary on the list are survival needs, such as food, water, and rest. Once these needs are met, however, there are higher needs, such as love and belonging, respect, status, freedom, fulfillment, and life purpose.

We all have our own set of universal needs, unique to us as individuals. But for understanding universal needs, many people turn to Maslow's hierarchy of needs, put together by American psychologist Abraham Maslow in 1943. Presented as a pyramid, the hierarchy ranks human needs from the most basic to higher needs having to do with self-fulfillment.

At the lowest and most basic level, for instance, are physical needs like food, water, and sleep. The next level underlines the need for safety and security. Love and belonging is the next level. The fourth level is self-esteem—we gravitate toward situations that enhance our sense of self-worth. At the top is self-actualization—the need to fulfill our greatest potential.

Universal needs are very powerful because they drive your behavior. Suffering in your life, on the other hand, occurs when you have needs that aren't being met.

You can solve many of life's challenges by figuring out which of your needs are not being met—then meeting them. Let's say you lose your job, for example. Afterward, you're depressed. This may be because you've lost such needs as *status, security,* or even *social connection.* Once you meet those needs, you'll feel better, with an optimistic outlook on your future.

Maybe right now something feels off in your life. Or you're down or anxious. Perhaps there's just something missing, but you can't put your finger on it. Why?

The answer may lie in the fact that you have unmet needs. According to Maslow, if you're struggling with something like dissatisfaction, frustration, depression, anxiety, or even addiction, it may be because one or more of your universal needs are not being satisfied.

When this is going on, you're going to feel negative. Likewise, when your needs are being met, you'll feel positive.

Here's the deal: rather than dwell on whether there's something "wrong" with you, ask yourself: "Which of my needs is not being met right now?" This question unlocks the door to why you're feeling off. When you identify your unmet needs, you can do something about them.

Beyond your physical needs, such as food, water, and rest, here is a list of four categories of general needs, and specific needs within them. Look these over and select needs you know are unmet in your life. Then strategize ways to meet them.

Category 1: Safety—Financial Security, Protection, Health and Well-Being (Safety Against Illness and Injury), and Shelter

We all need safe places that let us lead our lives without undue worry or fear about our finances, security, health, or living conditions.

If any of these needs are not being met: Ask yourself whether anything in your world is causing you to feel insecure or unsafe. Then take action to change it. For example, perhaps you'd feel safer if you installed a security system in your home. Or if you don't feel secure in your current neighborhood, set a plan in motion to move elsewhere.

Or maybe you're anxious over being let go from your current job or you're dissatisfied with your place of employment. If worried or unhappy at work, then quit your BS job and go for something that really ignites your passion.

Maybe a close relative passed away from a preventable disease. You don't want to go down the same road, so you make big lifestyle changes that will guard you from illness in the future.

Category 2: Love and Belonging—Strong Relationships, a Close Family, or Being Part of a Group

Connection, which we cover in Chapters 5 and 10, has turned out to be a vital part of health and happiness—on par with exercise and nutrition. To fulfill these needs and enhance every corner of your life, it's vital to have friends, feel love and intimacy, and experience connectedness with others.

If any of these needs are not being met: Make time for your friends and family. Or work on making new friends. Are you in an intimate relationship but feeling disconnected? Communicate honestly and express what it is you need from your partner, or seek couples counseling.

Maybe you need to join a group that gives you a sense of belonging and companionship. Or do volunteer work for an organization you care about. Join a gym, take classes (or as we call them, camps), or network in a professional organization. There are unlimited ways to get connected.

Category 3: Esteem—Acceptance by Others, Recognition, Respect, or Prestige

Each one of us needs to fulfill our top potential, achieve some sort of status in the world, strive to be relevant, and be recognized for our contributions.

If any of these needs are not being met: You deserve to live your life to the fullest—and the potential to do so is within your reach. Yet a lot of people experience only a fraction of their potential because they've never realized that they matter or are even aware of the impact they've already made on the world around them. Are you in that group?

Try this exercise: Imagine that today is your hundredth birthday, and the newspaper in your town is going to publish a big feature story on your life. Write your story as you'd like to see it printed. What accomplishments will you list? How would you describe your contributions? How did you influence the lives of others? What has been really important in your life?

Be honest and don't hold back. List significant milestones—recognitions, awards, contributions, qualifications, promotions, giving up any bad habits, and surviving all the rough patches in life. You have skills and strengths that helped you overcome obstacles, difficulties, trials, and challenges.

After you do this exercise, you'll realize the profound impact you had on the world around you, that you've made a huge difference, and that you touched lives in ways you hadn't realized.

Category 4: Self-Actualization—Realization of Your Potential, Accomplishment, Creativity, or Having a Higher Purpose in Life

You must feel that your life has genuine meaning—that you're a part of something greater than yourself—or it won't have the gravity to pull you through challenging times.

If any of these needs are not being met: You can find meaning in big things and small things. It's not that complicated! Start a family. Support a cause you believe in. Find faith or a belief system. Experience joy in small things like being out in nature, sipping tea, breathing fresh air, meditating, or watching sunrises and sunsets. When you learn to appreciate the little things, you'll find meaning everywhere you go.

Once you meet your specific needs, you'll realize you have more power over your own life—in your relationships, your profession, your community, and more—than you ever realized.

FOCUS ON PURPOSE AND PASSION.

A while back, there was a time when we both lost our professional anchors—the Giants contract and a good corporate job. We both needed a new calling—a new purpose in life. We eventually discovered it—helping people achieve inner and outer strength. It was pure satisfaction and a fulfillment we had never experienced in our prior careers.

Whether you're crushing life right now or at rock bottom, we want you to clearly define your purpose. Purpose is your why—why you get up in the morning, even when the day looks bleak, you're still sleepy, or you know the stuff ahead is going to be tough. It is grounded in the people you love and would never let down. Those people are your reason for living.

With purpose, you know what you want out of life. You also enjoy better physical, mental, and spiritual health. It lowers your odds of chronic disease and mental disorders. Lots of research has found that a purposeful life can even help you live longer!

So, how do you find that purpose?

Here's an exercise to help you identify your purpose. Simply ask yourself the following series of questions and write down your answers:

1. Who do I love the most in this world?
2. Who is most important to me?
3. Who have I shared my happiest moments and experiences with?

Besides your purpose, there are your passions. To identify your passions, look at what you're good at, asking people who know you best to get their opinions on your passions, or thinking about what brings you happiness and joy. And here's an exercise to help you identify your passion.

1. What values and beliefs am I unwilling to negotiate with?
2. What makes me feel fulfilled?
3. What is my calling? (not my career)
4. What would I wake up and pursue every day if money wasn't a consideration?

This exercise is neither complicated nor theoretical. It helps you focus on what you're living for so that you no longer have to wander aimlessly.

You know what you want and what you want to become. Your purpose is the compass that gets you there.

You want to create permanent change in your life. You want to forge lasting transformation. With the Believe strategy, you can reprogram your mind to believe that you can attract anything you want in life. No more starting over. No more New Year's resolutions. No more "dieting down" for some event or season. This strategy helps you live on your own terms— believing is the definition of happiness. Do what you want, when you want, with whom you want. Learn the power of permanent transformation when you apply this strategy.

CHAPTER 8

NUTRITION IS CRITICAL, BUT EASIER THAN YOU THINK (THE BURN 10-MINUTE MEAL PLAN)

MAKING SMALL CHANGES IS A KEY PART OF OUR NUTRITION PROGRAM. IT teaches you to become more food aware and how you can easily lose weight without making drastic changes. Eventually you can get off junk food, stop going on crazy diets and starving yourself, or taking appetite suppressants as Morgan once did. For a few days or even weeks, these fads may seem to work. You lose a few pounds, feel good about it, but soon you get tired of eating like that. The scale goes back up and won't slide back down. Now you're faced with those pounds to lose and you feel like crap because you failed.

We're going to ask you to stop with all that and roll with a new way of eating and thinking. Change things up. Get rid of thinking you're on a "diet"—it's blocking you from living the kind of life you want, and it's let you down. Start thinking of food as fuel and nourishment and cement this new mindset in your brain. If you think otherwise, you're screwed. We mean it! Open up your mind to doing food and nutrition differently.

Different is good. The only way to improve your future health is to do something different today.

We're here to help you change things up, and we're going to make it easy for you. We've created a nutritional eating plan that leads to permanent, positive changes.

Here's how it works. You start with a few simple changes that are healthier, give you more energy, and help you fit into clothes that make you feel like a million bucks. Then you move on to a total eating plan—the Burn 10-Minute Meal Plan—for breakfast, lunch, dinner, and snacks. We'll be with you through this entire process, answering your questions and keeping you motivated. We know you can do it.

You don't have to learn to like raw broccoli or bland baked chicken breasts either. You don't have to choke down dry, tasteless rice cakes. Instead, you get to enjoy delicious meals that can be made in ten minutes or less. There are fifty recipes to choose from.

While enjoying these meals, you'll be retraining yourself to *love* wholesome foods—lean proteins, fresh fruits and vegetables, natural carbohydrates, healthy fats, and more. Plus, there are so many genuinely tasty, healthy things to enjoy these days, and more and more nutritious options when eating out.

You can do all this without denying or depriving yourself, and if you do it with intention and awareness, even though it takes effort, we promise you it will pay off, although it's by no means easy. The most challenging thing you can do in life is to change a bad or unhealthy habit. But when you do find your *purpose* in life, healthy eating habits become easy because you've been faced with the pain of not achieving your blueprint in life. The most consistent force in humans is to stay consistent with who they believe they are.

SMALL NUTRITIONAL WINS

If you want to make permanent changes in your eating habits, you've got to start small. Sometimes, we get frustrated because the end result seems so far away, and we forget to honor the small successes on the journey. This is where "small wins" enter the picture. It's a framework to help you make, and be proud of, the small, achievable wins along the way.

We start you off with keeping a short three-to-seven-day food log, in which you zero in on what you're eating in terms of nutrients and calories, and whether your current diet is lacking in anything. This is an important tool. It flexes your awareness muscle. Awareness is a big leap toward change.

Next, for one or two weeks, we want you to make just one of the five small changes in your eating habits. We call these "small wins," and they lead to big, lasting change. You can't develop great health habits overnight. Lasting change requires a gradual approach. If you try to bite off more than you can chew—like tackling big, dramatic lifestyle changes—chances are you'll get discouraged and feel defeated. And discouragement and defeat are no longer options.

Repeat the same habit—a small change—with success for three weeks or more before moving on to the next small win. Have patience and focus on one tiny win at a time.

So—here are the five small changes we want you to make. Start with these and build from here.

Win #1: 100 Grams of Protein Daily

Protein does so much for your body. It acts as an enzyme for chemical reactions, repairs and builds muscle tissue, burns fat, regulates hormones, and so much more.

We all have different protein requirements, but a good target to start with and hit each day is 100 grams. If you're very active, you may need more, while less active people can do with less.

It's simple to tally up around 100 grams in a day from common foods. For example:

One large egg—6 grams
6 ounces plain Greek yogurt—17 grams

1 tablespoon peanut butter—4 grams

One 6.5-ounce can tuna—31 grams

½ cup cottage cheese—12 grams

One 3-ounce chicken breast—24 grams

½ cup cooked black beans—8 grams

Total—102 grams of protein

Win #2: Remove Added Sugar

Work toward zero grams of added sugar. But understand that there is a distinction between added sugar and natural sugar. Natural sugar is sugar that's naturally present in such food as fruits and dairy. Added sugar is just as it sounds—sugar that has been plunked into food during processing to sweeten or enhance the flavor.

Among the worst sources of added sugar are refined, processed carbohydrates (usually in packaged goods). Avoid this sweet stuff as much as possible. It causes a lot of harm due to its effect on blood sugar, insulin, and weight. In fact, a report in the *European Journal of Preventive Cardiology* noted that eating too much added sugar causes large fat deposits to form around the heart and in the abdomen—a huge risk factor for heart attacks.

Here are examples of added-sugar foods to ditch:

- Sugar-sweetened drinks, such as regular soft drinks, flavored coffees, sports drinks, energy drinks, and juice drinks
- Candy
- Commercially baked goods (cookies, cakes, pies, pastries, toaster tarts, doughnuts, and so forth)
- Sugary cereals, including sweetened instant oatmeal
- Sweetened dairy products (such as ice cream and flavored yogurt)
- Microwaveable dinners like sweet-and-sour chicken
- Jams and jellies
- Barbecue sauce
- Ketchup

Win #3: Increase Your Hydration

Here's one of the simplest adjustments you can make: drinking more water daily. Daily hydration can increase your metabolism up to 30 percent (particularly if you're already dehydrated) with the goal of working up to at least half your bodyweight in ounces of water.

Besides revving up your metabolism, staying hydrated helps you in other ways. Adequate hydration:

- Suppresses your appetite by taking up space in your tummy
- Helps your body flush out toxins that can interfere with good health
- Increases lipolysis, the process by which your body burns fat for energy
- Is good for cardiovascular health
- Boosts energy
- Enhances brainpower
- Improves digestion
- Lubricates your joints

How can you drink more water? Rather than the worn-out advice "drink eight glasses a day," we've got a better idea. Create two "hydration events" daily. Set aside five minutes twice a day to focus on drinking the necessary amount of water—which is, at minimum, half your bodyweight in ounces. Do this and you won't have to be concerned about staying hydrated or taking so many bathroom breaks.

Make your hydration events a part of your day. Make them nonnegotiable and eventually habitual, like brushing your teeth.

For a pop of flavor in your water, add cucumber slices, whole fresh berries, or a squeeze of grapefruit, orange, lemon, or lime. Lemon water is our favorite because it reduces inflammation, supports liver function, cleanses the body, and flushes out toxins.

In addition to your hydration events, enjoy other beverages too:

- Black coffee, known to fight inflammation in the body and provide antioxidants, B vitamins, and several minerals

- Unsweetened tea, which can support heart health because it is high in antioxidants
- Green juice, which contains various plant nutrients and chlorophyll, which strengthens your immune system, tames inflammation, and increases red blood cell production to boost oxygen flow throughout your body

Win #4: Control Your Alcohol Intake

Make your target no more than zero to four alcoholic beverages a week. Do your best to not spread them out to multiple days per week. Here's why: When booze enters your body, your liver says: "Whoa, alcohol is coming in. Let's stop burning everything else [like body fat], and burn alcohol instead." So, basically, fat-burning grinds to a halt while the liver shifts its metabolic gears to burn off the alcohol. Also, alcohol contains a lot of sugar, which can be easily converted to body fat, and in excess can damage such organs as the heart and liver. You also have to consider the fact that alcohol can be addictive and thus very destructive to a person's happiness, success, and overall mental health. We want to experience life through a clear, unfoggy lens, and alcohol is the number one disrupter to your worldview. Alcoholics have trouble finding their purpose in life—getting drunk leaves them feeling depressed and unfulfilled.

Win #5: Become Calorie Accountable

Calories are your source of energy and will ultimately determine the energy balance in your body. In an energy surplus, you gain weight (either fat or muscle or both). In an energy deficit, you reduce body fat.

How many calories and macronutrients do you need each day?

That number depends on so many factors—your age, gender, height, current weight, body composition, activity level, overall health, and fitness goals, among others. But, generally speaking, the requirements look like this:

Women—1,500 to 2,500 calories

Men—2,000 to 3,000 calories

The beauty of the Burn 10-Minute Meal Plan is that we do all the calorie counting and macro calculations for you. You really do not have to count; just follow the plan, and you automatically stay "food aware"—that is, within the range of calories for your goals.

These small wins lead to the most amazing thing: a chain reaction begins. When you eat well, you feel better, which can motivate you to move. The more you move, the more your body craves healthier foods, protein, and a more challenging workout. Before you know it, this chain reaction has you building muscle and feeling stronger, and permeates the rest of your life.

Kick Your Bad Eating Habits!

Ever wondered why you snack on chips or eat dessert every night when you know fruit would be better for you?

The answer lies in our *neuroassociations*. Neuroassociations are the links created between what you experience and the emotions and thoughts connected with it.

When you do or feel something the first time, your brain forms a thin neural pathway—a neuroassociation. Its purpose is to help you remember the particular activity, emotion, or behavior in the future. For instance, if you touch something hot and burn yourself, a new neuroassociation is formed, and it will prevent you from burning yourself again.

Repeating an activity, behavior, or emotion strengthens neuroassociations, however. Habits form as a result, and some can be tough to break.

Behind the formation of these pathways—and, thus, our behavior— is the desire to *avoid pain* and *seek pleasure*. The reason we make poor decisions or engage in bad habits boils down to pain and pleasure neuroassociations. Have a junk food habit? It can be traced back to the fact that you get pleasure from munching on crunchy chips but associate pain with snacking on veggies instead.

But if you want to break your neuroassociations, there's a way out!

Make the pain of your habits real. Imagine vividly into the future about how disgusted you feel about yourself because of your poor eating habits. The fat rolls around your waist. Sitting on the couch unable to move. Embarrassment at wearing baggy clothes. Doubling your weight in a few years. The pain of being alone because people may have left you, because you failed to love yourself enough to make a small series of changes years ago.

Do this every day for twenty-one days. Feel the same feelings. Let them intensify. Imagine these situations so clearly that they become real to you.

This will reprogram your mind and associate your feelings and projected behaviors with a loss of love—which subconsciously forces you to change so as to protect that love.

This exercise helps you reach a pain threshold, in which your brain signals to you: "I can't stand this anymore; it's unbearable. Do something!"

You'll begin to stop engaging in the sabotaging behaviors, and those strong neuroassociations get weaker and weaker. Eventually, the bad habits fade and disappear.

On the other hand, as healthy changes take hold in your life and health, you begin to form positive neuroassociations. Examples: The emotions you feel when you walk on the beach in a bathing suit, feeling good about your healthy body. Or the thrill of being able to dance, run, and work out with lots of energy. Or feeling mentally sharp after sticking to better nutrition habits.

Understanding your neuroassociations can help you understand why you do the things you do and prevent you from making unhealthy decisions in the future.

HOW THE BURN 10-MINUTE MEAL PLAN WORKS

Small wins never stop and there is no time frame. You're tackling your small wins (one at a time) until you've mastered that habit and it has become a routine. Then you move on to the next small win. You'll want to fuel your body when working out hard—so getting the appropriate amount of calories into your body within a twenty-four-hour period is vital. We aren't going to tell you when to eat, what to eat, how to eat it, or any other specific information that likely won't apply to you. Most everyone far overestimates how complex a healthy eating strategy is. Let's keep things simple: we want you to consume all your calories in a twenty-four-hour period and work on mastering the five small wins over time.

What will you eat? Proteins, such as meat, poultry, fish, shellfish, and eggs, and dairy foods, such as cheese and yogurt. Virtually all veggies and many fruits. Plenty of healthy fats from avocados, nuts, and good oils. Even carbs, such as sprouted bread, sweet potatoes, and winter squashes. Can you dine out? Absolutely!

You get to personalize your daily plan by mixing and matching your meals and snacks. You build that plan from fifty different delicious recipes.

Simply look over the recipes. Then select one breakfast, one lunch, one dinner, and snacks from the list, and you have your daily meal plan. Each recipe is listed with its calorie and macro content. You don't have to count anything in the recipes; we've done that for you.

There are five calorie plans: 1,500, 1,800, 2,000, 2,500, and 3,000, each designed for your individual needs and goals—weight loss, weight maintenance, muscle gain, or fueling higher-performance workouts.

As an illustration, if you want to eat 1,500 calories a day, look over the list of recipes, and choose those with calories that add up to a daily count of 1,500. For example, choose a breakfast with 350 calories, a lunch with 400 calories, and dinner with 450 calories, plus two snacks totaling 300 (150 each), and you have just created your 1,500-calorie meal plan for the day. It's that easy—and keeps you food aware.

We created sample daily meal plans for you, but you have the freedom to select different meals every day or repeat your favorite meals. If you love oatmeal every day for breakfast, then go for it!

As part of staying accountable and aware, we want you to track calories and nutrients for three full days every ninety days, using an app like

MyFitnessPal or Lose It! If you create your own recipes for the plan or eat out a lot, you can log in their nutrients and dishes too. Of course, these apps help you stay calorie accountable as well. And some apps have weekly health tests that give you insight on your habits and identify potential areas for improvement.

If you take time to track this information, you'll get a better understanding of what you're actually eating and drinking on a routine basis.

Also, make meal prep a habit. Designate one day a week as your meal prep day. We like to do this on Sundays because it's the most relaxed day of the week. You'll prep and cook the meals you choose from the list. Once everything is prepared or cooked, separate the meals into containers and keep them in your fridge. Before you leave in the morning, grab the meals and put them in your bag or a small cooler. The beauty of meal prep is that healthy food is accessible; we're less tempted to eat junk food from a vending machine or fast-food place. A meal prep routine provides you with convenient, healthy options.

THE BURN 10-MINUTE MEAL PLANS

These complete, modular meals provide an easy way to help you achieve your nutritional goals. Remember, you don't have to count anything. Just follow these meals, or choose your own, and you'll be food aware effortlessly, and you'll be on your way to great nutrition and health. (The recipes are in Appendix B.)

MEAL PLAN—1,500				
Use this plan if you are a woman who works out most days of the week and wants to reduce body fat.				
Meal	**Calories**	**Protein (g)**	**Carbohydrates (g)**	**Fat (g)**
Meal 1				
AM Shake: 1 After-burn shake + 5mg creatine*	110	23	2	1
Greek Yogurt Par-fait with Fruit	290	20	36	4
Meal 2				
Classic Chicken and Sweet Potato	359	48	33	5
Meal 3				
Bison and Sweet Potato Mash	498	42	23	26
Snack 1				
Cinnamon Oat Muffin	164	15	17	5
Snack 2				
Afterburn Coffee	192	24	6	10
Totals	**1,613**	**172**	**117**	**51**

* Creatine monohydrate is a combination of amino acids that improve performance, help fuel muscles to create lean muscle mass, encourage fat loss, and provide a faster next-day recovery. When taken daily, creatine will get you through those last reps and that next-day soreness so that you can get back to your workout.

MEAL PLAN—1,800				
Use this plan if you are a man who works out most days of the week and wants to reduce body fat, or a woman who wants to maintain her weight.				
Meal	**Calories**	**Protein (g)**	**Carbohydrates (g)**	**Fat (g)**
Meal 1				
AM Shake: 1 Afterburn shake + 5mg creatine	110	23	2	1
Green Omelet with Ezekiel Bread	428	38	45	10
Meal 2				
Chicken Kale Salad and Lemon Vinaigrette	355 105	37 1	26 27	16 0
Meal 3				
Beef and Quinoa Baked Burrito	315	22	28	13
Snack 1				
½ cup of hummus spread on cucumber slices (1 cup)	307 16 119	20 1 0	26 4 28	24 0 0
Snack 2				
Greek Yogurt Parfait with Fruit	290	20	36	4
Totals	**1,821**	**161**	**167**	**68**

MEAL PLAN—2,000				
Use this plan if you are a man who works out most days of the week and wants to reduce body fat, or a woman who wants to maintain her weight or develop muscle.				
Meal	Calories	Protein (g)	Carbohydrates (g)	Fat (g)
Meal 1				
AM Shake: 1 Afterburn shake + 5mg creatine	110	23	2	1
4 egg whites, scrambled, and 2 slices Ezekiel bread	229	22	31	1
Meal 2				
Apple Walnut Chicken Salad	441	39	25	54
Meal 3				
Lean Turkey Dinner with Chocolate Chip Cookie Dough Pudding	394 239	38 30	36 28	12 5
Snack 1				
Mint Milkshake	369	28	41	13
Snack 2				
Apples and Peanut Butter	202	21	30	2
Totals	**1,984**	**201**	**193**	**88**

MEAL PLAN—2,500				
Use this plan if you are an active man who wants to maintain his weight, or even gain muscle weight. It features an additional meal so as to bump up daily calories.				
Meal	**Calories**	**Protein (g)**	**Carbohydrates (g)**	**Fat (g)**
Meal 1				
AM Shake: 1 Afterburn shake + 5mg creatine	110	23	2	1
No-Bake Oats	300	24	40	8
Meal 2				
Bison and Sweet Potato Mash, with Protein Brownie Mug Cake	498 190	42 27	23 15	26 4
Meal 3				
Mustard Salmon with Grilled Asparagus, with a medium baked sweet potato	326 100	42 2	11 23	12 0
Meal 4				
Chicken Fajita Bowl, with Protein Power Cups	292 100	26 16	38 2	6 16
Snack 1				
Chocolate Banana Smoothie	341	28	33	14
Snack 2				
*Snack pack: 1 large hard-boiled egg, a handful of almonds, and 1 medium peach	77 164 58	6 6 1	0 6 15	5 14 0
Totals	**2,556**	**243**	**208**	**106**

*Generic snack

MEAL PLAN—3,000				
This plan is generally best for male athletes performing at high levels of intensity and who desire to gain muscle. It features an additional meal so as to bump up daily calories.				
Meal	**Calories**	**Protein (g)**	**Carbohydrates (g)**	**Fat (g)**
Meal 1				
AM Shake: 1 Afterburn shake + 5mg creatine	110	23	2	1
4 egg whites, scrambled, and 2 slices Ezekiel bread	229	22	31	1
Meal 2				
Chicken Avocado Spinach Salad, with Protein Brownie Mug Cake	377 190	33 27	15 15	21 4
Meal 3				
Lean Spaghetti and Meatballs	360	34	18	17
Meal 4				
Coconut-Crusted Chicken Fingers, with Protein-Packed Cauliflower Mash	270 320	39 32	7 21	19 15
Snack 1				
Chocolate Banana Smoothie	341	28	33	14
Snack 2				
Stuffed 'Bellos, with Afterburn Coffee	320 192	48 24	9 6	10 10
Snack 3				
*Snack pack: 2 large hard-boiled eggs, a handful of almonds	154 164	12 6	0 6	10 14
Totals	**3,027**	**328**	**163**	**136**

*Generic snack

THE THREE-QUESTION TEST

As you'll see in our meal plan, we have one common denominator—simplicity. In a busy, grab-and-go society, the complexity of healthy eating can be overwhelming. With macros, deficits, and the effect of certain foods on metabolism and blood sugar, there are countless quantifiable variables you could use to measure. It's so darn confusing, even for us. In the spirit of simplicity, we created another easy way to keep yourself food aware. Just ask and answer the following three questions:

1. Do I have more energy today than yesterday?
2. Do I feel leaner today than yesterday?
3. Am I proud of the food choices I made yesterday?

If you can answer yes to all three, then you know that whatever your scale says is irrelevant. If your answer is no, then you have some adjustments to make. The key to holding yourself accountable in this fashion is to eliminate judgment for trying. The act of trying and failing moves you closer and closer to success without shame, doubt, or guilt.

THE POWER OF SWAPS

We love food swaps, and so will you! Food swaps are healthy food substitutions that mimic higher-calorie, low-nutrition foods, and many of our recipes use them. Swaps are dense in nutrients and have higher amounts of vitamins and minerals than their normal counterparts. Using swaps helps you feel more satisfied, and you don't feel that you're giving anything up. We've pulled together a comprehensive list of our favorite swaps from proteins to carbs to fats and everything in between. They'll help you make great nutritional changes easily, without added stress.

You'll love how many simple food substitutions there are and how easy they are to fit in. And the best part? Most times, you'll never be able to tell the difference.

TOP SWAP-OUTS—For Breakfast		
Eat This	**Not This**	**Why It's Better**
1 cup steel-cut oats or rolled oats	½ cup granola	These oats have twice the whole grains and half the sodium. Plus, granola is loaded with sugar.
2 slices Ezekiel bread or toast	1 plain bagel	Ezekiel bread is a sprouted-grain product. It is easier to digest and contains more nutrients than a plain bagel, and half the calories and sodium.
1 cinnamon raisin Ezekiel English muffin	1 blueberry muffin	Sprouted grains are easier on digestion. Plus, this cinnamon muffin satisfies your sweet tooth with far less sugar and fewer calories.
2 egg whites and 1 whole egg	3 whole eggs	Eggs are an excellent source of protein and healthy fats. Mixing egg whites with whole eggs is a great way to balance your fat intake.
4 ounces lean ground turkey	4 breakfast sausage links	Season the ground turkey with fennel, paprika, garlic, sage, and pure maple syrup to get the breakfast sausage flavor but without added preservatives and sodium.
½ cup fresh berries	1 cup juice	Eat fruit, rather than drink it. Juices are high in sugar and devoid of the natural fiber you find in whole fruits.

TOP SWAP-OUTS—For Lunch		
Eat This	**Not This**	**Why It's Better**
Turkey lettuce wraps	Turkey and cheese sub	Cut out the overprocessed cheese and white sub roll and swap nitrate-free deli turkey with fresh tomatoes and onions wrapped in a romaine lettuce leaf. It's far fewer calories and just as satisfying.
BLAT (bacon, lettuce, avocado, and tomato)	BLT (bacon, lettuce, and tomatoes)	Nitrate-free bacon (or turkey bacon) and Ezekiel bread are a great way to save calories on this classic. Swap out mayo for mashed avocado and you're all set.
Ground turkey, sweet potatoes, and broccoli	Frozen turkey, mashed potatoes, and green beans	Ground turkey breast served with mashed sweet potatoes and steamed broccoli makes a hearty, healthy meal, without the huge calorie and starch price tag.
Fresh greens, nuts, seeds, grilled chicken, and vinaigrette	Salad with ranch dressing and croutons	Ranch dressing and buttery croutons turn a light lunch into a calorie bomb. Use fresh greens and veggies and top them with 4 ounces of grilled chicken. Add nuts and seeds for crunch and dress with a lemon vinaigrette.
Apple butter and strawberries sandwich	Peanut butter and jelly sandwich	Change up the classic PB & J sandwich by using an Ezekiel English muffin with apple butter and sliced fresh strawberries.

TOP SWAP-OUTS—For Lunch		
Eat This	**Not This**	**Why It's Better**
Quinoa taco salad	Restaurant burrito	Skip the Mexican takeout line. Season ground beef with low-sodium taco seasoning and combine with grilled onions and peppers, served over quinoa. Top with salsa and almond cheese and enjoy.
Tuna salad	Takeout tuna salad	Tuna (or chicken) coated in mashed avocado and lime juice makes the perfect sandwich or lettuce topper.

TOP SWAP-OUTS—For Dinner		
Eat This	**Not This**	**Why It's Better**
Classic Chicken and Sweet Potato Meal	Chicken cutlet, mashed potatoes, and veggies	This meal is packed with lean protein and veggies to energize your body without the heavy starch and extra calories.
Spaghetti squash and meatballs	Spaghetti and meatballs	Make your meatballs with ground chicken or turkey and serve over spaghetti squash, a nutrient-rich alternative to pasta.
London broil steak and potatoes	Rib-eye steak and fries	London broil is a lean cut of meat. Serve it grilled with boiled red-skinned potatoes and asparagus for a complete meal.
BBQ pork tenderloin	BBQ pulled pork	Swap out fatty Boston butt for a lean pork tenderloin. Make your own BBQ sauce without all the added sugar.
Coconut-Crusted Chicken Fingers	Chicken nuggets	Ditch the heavy breading and unhealthy fats from deep-fried nuggets. Replace them with lean tenders coated in egg whites, and "breaded" with coconut flakes and crushed almonds.
Grilled Chicken Parm and Zucchini Pasta	Chicken Parmesan dinner	Sauté spiralized zucchini with garlic and cherry tomatoes to make a fresh sauce. Top with grilled chicken and freshly grated Parmesan cheese.
Chicken and Cauliflower "Fried Rice"	Takeout chicken with fried rice	Cauliflower rice is the perfect rice substitute. Add some stir-fried veggies and season with coconut aminos.

TOP SWAP-OUTS—Everyday Substitutions	
Eat This	**Not This**
Quinoa	White rice
Ezekiel bread	Whole wheat bread
Mashed cauliflower	Mashed potatoes
Mashed avocado	Mayonnaise
Oven-baked sweet potato fries	French fries
Spaghetti squash, spiralized vegetables	White pasta
Stevia in the Raw	Sugar and artificial sweeteners
Coconut aminos	Soy sauce
Coconut milk	Coffee creamer
Brown rice pasta	White pasta
Nut milk	Dairy milk
Cauliflower crust	Pizza crust
Coconut oil, olive oil, grapeseed oil	Butter, canola, or vegetable oil
Himalayan pink salt	Table salt
Lettuce wraps	Tortillas
Steel-cut or rolled oats	Instant oatmeal

SUCCESSFUL GROCERY SHOPPING

Good nutrition starts at the grocery store—with a list. To do that, create a shopping list based on the meals you've planned for the week. Organize your list by store section for quick and easy shopping, and bring the list with you when you go to the supermarket.

Everyone's shopping list will differ according to what is planned for the week. The following is a generic shopping list you can use as a model to create your own.

Dairy, Fats & Oils	Protein	Vegetables	Fruits
For cooking:	*Seafood*	*Squash*	*Apples*
Animal fats	(Wild-caught, not	Acorn, butternut,	Red Delicious
Clarified butter	farm-raised)	pumpkin, spa-	Granny Smith
Extra-virgin	Shellfish	ghetti, and winter	*Berries*
olive oil	Salmon	*Bell Peppers*	Blackberries, blue-
Grapeseed oil	Haddock	All colors	berries, raspber-
Sunflower oil	Tuna	*Cruciferous*	ries, strawberries
Coconut oil	Cod	*Vegetables*	*Melons*
(unrefined)	Mahi-mahi	Broccoli	Cantaloupe,
For eating:	*100% Grass-Fed*	Brussels sprouts	honeydew,
Avocados	*and Organic*	Cabbage	watermelon
Olives	Beef, bison, lamb,	Cauliflower	*Others*
Coconut flakes	elk, venison	*Greens*	Banana
(unsweetened)	*Pastured and*	Spinach, kale,	Cherries
Cheese (feta or	*Organic*	beet, mustard,	Grapes
goat)	Pork, rabbit	collard	Grapefruit
Milk (almond or	*Pastured and*	*Lettuce*	Kiwi
coconut)	*Organic Poultry*	All varieties	Lemon
Nuts (almonds,	Chicken, turkey,	*Mushrooms*	Lime
cashews,	duck, Cornish hen,	All varieties	Mango
hazelnuts,	pheasant, etc.	*Root Vegetables*	Orange
Macadamia,	*Processed Meats*	Beets, carrots,	Papaya
pecans, pistachios,	(Grass-fed/pas-	jicama, parsnips,	Peach
walnuts	teurized organic	rhubarb, rutabaga,	Pear
Nut butters	and nitrate-free)	turnip	Plum
(almond,	Bacon, sausage,	*Others*	Pomegranate
sunflower)	organic deli	Artichokes	Tangerine
Yogurt (Greek,	meat, etc.	Asparagus	
almond, coconut)	*Eggs & Liquid Egg*	Cucumbers	
	Whites	Green beans	
	(cage-free and/or	Radishes	
	organic)	Snow peas/sugar	
		snap beans	
		Sweet potato	
		Zucchini	
		Yellow beans	
		Tomatoes	
		Celery	
		Onions	

Canned Goods	Condiments/ Spices	Grains/Legumes	Sweets/Baking
Beans (all varieties) Beets Broth (organic chicken, beef, tur- key, or vegetable) Preserves (no added sugar) Tuna/salmon (wild-caught) Tomato sauce/ paste Salsa (organic) Sun-dried tomatoes Artichoke hearts Pumpkin	*All Herbs & Spices* Avoid seasoning mixes Organic ketchup Mustards *Extracts* Vanilla, almond, peppermint Chipotle hot pep- per (jarred) Horseradish Tabasco	All varieties Ezekiel bread, wraps, pita, and English muffins Brown rice Quinoa Steel-cut oatmeal	Stevia in the Raw Raw honey Dark chocolate or cacao chips (organic) Pure maple syrup Coconut sugar crystals Baking soda Almond/coconut flour

CAN YOU ORDER OUT?

Definitely! You do not need to sabotage your social life to stay healthy. Eating out and eating in can coexist by keeping a few guidelines in mind:

Sit-Down Restaurants. Your best bets here are to order a protein-based entrée, such as steak, chicken, or seafood, accompanied by a salad, vegetables, or sweet potato. Limit your alcohol intake, because when alcohol is present, the body starts storing the rest of food as fat. Avoid the bread basket too. It's full of starch and empty calories.

Fast-Food Establishments. Are these the best places to eat out? Not really, but you can make healthy choices here anyway. Always opt for grilled selections, for example. If you love burgers, eat only half the bun. And yes, even fast-food places have great salads. Another of our recommendations is found at Starbucks—the Egg White Bites. Just use your nutritional common sense and you'll make healthy choices. Chipotle is another go-to favorite for us.

On-the-Road Meals. We keep resealable bags in our car, called "snack packs," that typically contain protein bars, apples, cashews, beef jerky, and packets of almond or peanut butter.

A key to successful healthy eating starts the night before. You should always select tomorrow's meals today. Then wake up the next day with the reminder that—yes, you're worth it! So be good to your body with healthy nutrition at every meal, and your body will be good to you—especially in terms of inner and outer strength. If you love yourself like this, you'll see what's possible for you, and great health will be yours and something you very much deserve.

CHAPTER 9

ACHIEVE WHAT YOUR HEART DESIRES

J ESSIE LEARNED THROUGH LOSS AND HARDSHIP THAT YOU REACH YOUR destination with a road map—dotted not only with your goals, but also with the steps required to achieve them. Here is her inspirational account.

From our Kenosha, Wisconsin, camp, Jessie started her health and fitness journey in 2018, although she had been an athlete since childhood. As a mom of three, she was juggling the demands of motherhood but, in the quiet moments, dreamed of taking her strength and fitness, her whole life, to a higher level. "I wanted to love myself again," she recalls. "I wanted to feel proud of my body. I wanted to be confident in my own skin again."

After her first camp, Jessie was hooked. She felt empowered and proud. She showed up every day. "I craved the energy, the positivity, the high-fives, and the support and encouragement I received as soon as I walked through the door."

A year into her journey, Jessie set a goal for herself: to become a trainer. She had a specific reason that came from deep within her—and it wasn't to get more fit. Her "why," her passion for life, was rooted in her love for her late father. She lost him in 2022 from primary progressive aphasia, a rare form of dementia that affects the ability to communicate. He was only sixty-nine and a seventeen-time Ironman athlete who had competed in marathons, triathlons, and biking competitions until the disease robbed him of his motor skills. Raising her three children, Jessie realized that she wanted to pass on the same values of determination and strength to them while also fulfilling her own dream. She was determined to honor her late father's legacy.

"I got my passion for fitness from him. We shared that passion together. I work out every day for him."

Jessie set out to achieve small wins—actionable steps—to become a trainer. She first completed her personal training certification. She then interned as an assistant trainer, learning everything she could from one of our head trainers. That head trainer saw something in Jessie—that she could inspire people and was ready to be a full-fledged trainer. Today, she is now one of our head trainers.

From the beginning of her journey, Jessie knew that half-hearted efforts would not improve the future. It gets better by planning. And to plan, you must have goals rooted in a personal "why."

She brings this philosophy to work every day. "I always ask people, 'What is your "why"? Why are you doing this? If things get boring or you're ready to quit, what is the "why" that will keep you coming back?'"

Jessie's "why" is her dad. When she trains, she carries his passion and love for fitness in her heart and pours that into her camps. She competed in our Athlete Games twice and placed ninth in the Athlete Game Finals only five months after her father passed away. Her father's legacy lived on not only through her, but through the countless lives she's transformed.

"He would want me to keep pushing on and keep reaching for that next goal. So that's what I do. Through it all, I learned that I can do hard things and that I'm stronger than I ever thought. Whereas once I was a self-conscious, nervous woman in her forties, today I'm a confident trainer who knows her worth and the impact she has on others to reach their goals."

Jessie used our Achieve strategy successfully. It is a goal-setting system based on identifying your "North Star goals" in key categories of your life. These are large, aspirational goals designed around what you want your ideal life to look like in five to ten years, when you're feeling accomplished and successful. We then break those North Star goals down into specific, small actionable wins that change your day-to-day activities to get you to your North Star goals.

Before we dig into our North Star goal-setting system, we want to get clear on exactly why North Star goals are so powerful. Setting goals is like planning a road trip. You would never jump into your car and drive without first planning your route, right? Or without using a map or a GPS? How would you even get there?

Yet that's what a lot of people do—figuratively drive around with no clear route to a destination. They get lost. They end up back where they started. They stop trying and lose their enthusiasm. With this system, however, you'll get to your destination, and you'll start to think and act in ways that drive you toward success.

There are seven key steps involved in North Star goal-setting.

STEP 1. IDENTIFY YOUR NORTH STAR GOALS IN ONE OR MORE OF THESE CATEGORIES OF YOUR LIFE.

Start by pinpointing the area or areas of your life you'd like to transform. Look over the following list. We've given examples of what North Star goals might look like, but ultimately you'll want to personalize them to your own life.

+ Body
- Enjoy excellent physical, mental, and emotional health
- Be free from pain and illness
- Manage stress better
- Have higher levels of energy and vitality

+ Mind

- Develop a morning routine
- Practice daily gratitude
- Consider getting therapy
- Find joyful movement to relieve anxiety or depression
- Use positive self-talk

+ Emotions

- Find satisfaction with your life
- Stay connected to others
- Shift attention from negative emotions like anger to something more positive
- Pause and think before impulsively reacting when emotional
- Make peace with what you can't control

+ Spirit

- Speak to God or your Higher Power daily
- Spread love to your neighbors
- Help others in need
- Show compassion
- Promote peace
- Learn to forgive others

+ Relationships

- Create a plan in which you set forth your goals for your finances, housing, careers, children, and anything else that's important to achieve together
- Prioritize spending more time with your closest friends
- Plan more family activities

+ Time

- Spend more time working on your North Star goals
- Make choices to do only things that move you closer to success
- Figure out your priorities and reallocate more time to them

+ Work

- Add a second job that you enjoy in the evening or weekend if you can't quit your present job just yet

- Create a vision of the perfect job for you
- Change careers to an area of work that is more fulfilling and inspiring to you

+ Money

- Advance toward a job promotion or leadership position
- Acquire a certification
- Work toward greater personal development
- Commit to lifelong learning
- Develop a growth mindset
- Build a larger professional network
- Work with a financial adviser
- Consider where to invest your money

STEP 2. IDENTIFY YOUR "WHY."

After you select the category or categories, answer this question: Why do I want to transform myself in this area? Your answer to this question becomes the guiding light for every decision you make in your life and forms the basis for creating your North Star goals. When the "why" is clear, the "how" becomes easy.

As an example, if you told one of our trainers that you wanted to lose weight, that trainer will ask, "Why?"

As many people do, you might answer, "Because I want to be healthy and look better."

You'd get quizzed a little more. "And why do you want to be healthy and look better?"

You might respond something like this: "Why not? Doesn't everyone?"

At this point, the trainer will dig even deeper. "I get that, I really do. But what motivated you to come all the way down here, make an appointment with me, and want to dedicate all this time to losing weight?"

This line of questioning is designed to help you reflect deeply and come up with a reason specific to you. Maybe you had a parent who had died early because of an obesity-related disease. Or maybe your doctor told you that you have diabetes, and weight control is important. Perhaps you want to move around more easily and actively for your grandkids.

You then zero in on your true, deep-down motivation, and your whole attitude and approach will change. Up until that point, you had been looking for motivation in all the wrong places. Once you find your "why," you'll establish an emotional connection to what you care about most, cutting off any possibility, story, or excuse you've used in the past. Emotion creates motion. You'll be on your way to lasting change, and you won't have to keep making false starts anymore.

STEP 3. WRITE DOWN YOUR GOALS.

When you write down your goals by hand, recall that you trigger your reticular activating system (RAS) to start scanning for goal-achieving opportunities. With a specific target, the RAS works with your conscious mind to help you "see" opportunities that may have gone unnoticed. The RAS offers insights, searches past experiences for relevant intel, and provides inspiring ideas to be explored—all with the intent of giving you what you want and setting your course in a positive direction.

To start this process, take out a piece of paper, a pen, and a stopwatch, and get to work. Set the timer for ten minutes to do this step. Do it in solitude—no background music, no kids around, and no television or phone on—so that your mind is clear. Use the aforementioned examples of North Star goals as "thought starters" to get your juices flowing.

Now, write out every goal you can possibly think of for yourself on that piece of paper. Don't stop writing for ten minutes.

When finished, write a 10, 5, 3, or 1 next to each goal. The 10 is for ten years, 5 for five years, 3 for three years, and 1 for one year. You're predicting how much time you expect it to take to achieve particular goals. Transfer your goals and their respective time frame to a chart, categorized by ten years, five years, three years, and one year.

Look over your chart. There may be a few goals that are "nice to have," but you want to go for goals that you must have. Circle all your "must-haves"; erase or delete the rest.

Now, put them on your calendar; this makes them real. This is an ongoing list. We have hundreds of goals that we've set, both short- and long-term. But they're also flexible because setting goals is a process that changes over time. The goals you set five years ago might turn out to be different from the goals you want to set today. If you wake up one day and change your mind about your goals, it's perfectly okay to adjust them as long as you continually revisit your goals and work to update them.

STEP 4. ORGANIZE YOUR GOALS INTO ACTIONABLE STEPS.

We have observed that frequent, small achievements initiate a cycle of lasting change and create happiness. So break your long-term North Star goals into smaller chunks—even into steps for individual days, if possible. These steps represent potential daily wins that get you down the road to success.

Daily wins are powerful and have an equally powerful effect on your mind. A good example comes from the US Navy SEALs. To become a SEAL, trainees must swim an entire 50 meters underwater without taking a breath. It's not easy, and some trainees have a rough time with it.

One SEAL instructor observed that the trainees who struggled most with this requirement were the ones who were intimidated by it before they even attempted it. So the instructor told them to focus on executing each stroke individually instead of worrying about the full 50-meter stretch. Amazingly, the trainees performed much better than if they told themselves beforehand, "Oh no, I have to dive 50 meters." Small chunks equal big gains.

We call this process "reverse engineering" your goals. Basically, it involves working through a goal backward and creating small wins toward that goal.

Let's say one of your North Star goals is health related—such as losing 100 pounds in a year and keeping it off. That goal becomes manageable when you break it down into smaller, bite-size chunks.

Some examples of manageable daily activities:

- Stop drinking your calories in the form of sodas, commercial juices, or alcohol.
- Remove or cut down on added sugar.
- Stop buying junk food for others in your family.
- Drink more water.
- Attend a nutritional cooking class.
- Track your nutrient intake.
- Start the Burn 10-Minute Meal Plan.
- Make a habit of meal prep.
- Work out at least four to five times a week.
- Start building relationships with others so you can support one another in your weight management efforts.

Drilling down your North Star goal into actionable steps helps you move confidently toward achieving it.

Ask yourself: What are the most important five to ten steps I could take over the next twelve months to achieve my North Star goal? Write these down too.

Monitor yourself daily. Of the ten steps, how many of these are you actively pursuing? Do something every day to move toward your goals. One of the greatest forces in human nature is to stay consistent in moving toward your goals.

STEP 5. VISUALIZE YOUR GOALS.

The power behind visualizing your goals is that if you "see" your goal, you are more likely to achieve it. For example, you might visualize your clothes fitting better, tasting the delicious flavors in healthy foods you're eating, living in your dream home, or feeling how happy you are.

When we first started our careers and our family, we began to see how powerful visualization is. Every self-help guru and motivator on the planet talks about its importance. There's a reason that the most successful people in the world all believe in visualizing—it's because it works!

In fact, visualization is linked to a number of health benefits. Visualization can help you:

- Boost your athletic and exercise performance
- Ease symptoms of anxiety and depression
- Relax more
- Have more compassion for yourself and others
- Relieve pain
- Manage stress
- Enhance your sleep
- Improve your emotional and physical wellness
- Boost your self-confidence

So be very vivid in your imagination. What does your opportunity look like? What does it feel like? What sounds are associated with your desired outcome? What does it taste or smell like, if relevant? Make the visualization large too—as if it were projected on a huge movie screen. And—visualize the goal or opportunity as if you've already achieved it, and it is alive in your life. Do this repeatedly in your mind and opportunities are far more likely to present themselves.

Your brain can't always differentiate between what you've imagined and what has actually happened—a fact you can put to good use. Simply imagine your life as though you've already reached your goals. Close your eyes and envision yourself doing all the things you want to do, having the things you want to have, and becoming the person you want to be. When you see yourself getting what you want, your brain believes that you have already done those things. This makes it easier to achieve your goals in reality. It's been said that whatever you desire, it has already been placed in your path. Believe it!

By creating a clear and detailed image of what you want, you can focus your mind and energize your brain to work toward making it a reality. Whether you want to get healthy, save money, or start a business, visualizing your goals helps turn them into reality. Pretty amazing, right?

STEP 6. BRING YOUR NORTH STAR GOALS INTO VIEW AS YOU CLOSE IN ON THEM.

Researchers from the Stanford Graduate School of Business found that although you benefit from concentrating on small steps in the early stages of pursuing your goals, it's important to focus instead on the larger goal in the later stages. The reason is that small steps are achievable and great motivators early on. Then, once you close in on your big-picture goal, you become more motivated to attain it.

For example, say you've lost 30 pounds so far by choosing healthy foods each day or cutting out sugar. You probably feel assured that your final goal of losing 40 pounds can be reached. To stay motivated, shift your focus to the big 40-pound goal and what you need to do to push toward it.

Or take the example of marathoners. Early in a race they have their sights set on making it through various mile markers or checkpoints. But once they see the finish line, they focus on that and apply all their power and speed to making it.

Pursuing your goals is a dynamic process. What motivates you at the beginning is not the same as what helps you finish. So keep going! You're almost there.

STEP 7. STAY WITH IT!

Every single day, work on those steps and never quit. There's a cool story told about a high school basketball coach who wanted to inspire his players to stick with it through a tough season. He asked his team, "Did Michael Jordan ever quit?" The team responded, "No!" "Did Serena Williams ever give up?" "No," the team said. "Did Tom Brady ever give up?" Again, the players said, "No!" Finally, the coach said, "Did Elmer McAllister ever quit?"

Silence fell over the locker room. Then one player bravely spoke up, "Who's Elmer McAllister? We've never heard of him."

The coach replied, "Of course, you've never heard of him. He quit!"

This type of full-on perseverance—refusing to quit on your goals—is what helped Drew, from our Flower Mound, Texas, camp, defy the odds and create lasting change in his life.

"I've been living with severe arthritis pain in my joints most of my adult life, which greatly limits my mobility. A year ago, I started resistance training, but I was too afraid to lift more than 10 pounds at a time on any given exercise. I felt I could do more, and I wanted to feel stronger and less fragile."

After consulting with his doctor, Drew decided to work with a trainer who had experience with people having his condition. "I told him that my goal was to get stronger, but up until that point I had never imagined that I could because it would involve increasing weight. He explained to me that resistance training was an important therapy for people like me to relieve the joint pain and stiffness. Not exercising enough could actually make my joints stiffer and even more painful. That was the only thing he needed to say."

Drew first had to change his focus—from thinking that he could not lift a lot of weight to thinking that he could. Then he took actionable steps to get stronger, and he stuck with them.

"We got to work, making sure I lifted a little more each week. I gradually started lifting 15 pounds, then 25 pounds, 30 pounds, and more. It wasn't always easy. There were days when I just didn't want to try. But I did. I didn't quit. And my progress amazed me."

After six months and with permission from his doctor, Drew was bench-pressing 100 pounds!

"The increases in my strength and improvements in my ability were honestly beyond what I ever thought I could achieve. Feeling stronger is a completely new thing for me, and it makes me feel much better physically and emotionally. My confidence is through the roof."

Whatever your goals are, the willingness to "keep on keeping on" will determine your measure of success. So whatever you want, keep pushing a little each day, and you'll eventually get what you're after.

STEP 8. MEASURE YOUR NORTH STAR GOALS.

There's a familiar saying: "What gets measured gets managed." A lot of people who set goals measure their progress by how it feels. Don't rely on feeling; rely on numbers. The beauty of formulating a North Star goal into a number is that numbers don't lie. In building our business, we inserted numbers: more than six hundred franchises by 2024. That last number is key—by when. Always have a time in which you want to achieve your North Star goal.

Goal-setting is not something that you do once and then forget about it. So, periodically, check and review your progress toward your goals. Measure your goals by whether you complete them when you said you would. When you do this, you become even more aligned with your goals. You make them come alive by doing something about them.

As you go forward, don't let anyone influence how you decide to reach your goals. They might sound too big and lofty to them, but these are your goals. We believe in thinking big and shooting for the stars. Never let anyone tell you that you can't aim big. Other people might not be willing to do what it takes, but you're different and have higher aspirations. Go for them.

CHAPTER 10

CREATE YOUR CIRCLE
OF CONNECTION

S OCIAL CONNECTION IS A HUGE PREDICTOR OF A HAPPY LIFE—AND MAY even bring about healing. Samantha found connection at the gym during a brutal, scary time in her life. Her story is one of the most amazing accounts of healing and survival we have ever heard.

From playing soccer to track to volleyball and being a spin instructor, Samantha, from our Naples, Florida, camp, has been involved in health and fitness for as long as she can remember. Until she was twenty-six, she thought she was a healthy young woman: strong and in near-perfect shape. She worked out at the gym regularly and hardly missed a day.

Then, suddenly and without warning, came terrifying news: Samantha was diagnosed with breast cancer. "My world turned upside down. I couldn't believe at twenty-six years old, I had cancer and that I would have to go through chemo, lose my hair, and make gut-wrenching decisions about reproductive considerations. My husband and I wanted kids."

As it turned out, Samantha required a mastectomy without any need for chemo, radiation, or other treatments. "After about five months, I was all reconstructed, recovered, in the gym, and back to normal life. My husband and I thought this diagnosis was the most difficult thing that we would ever have to endure as a couple."

This was not to be. At age twenty-nine, Samantha experienced a cluster of strange symptoms: severe chills alternating with intense, boiling hot heat; loss of appetite; and no energy. She was also nearly thirty weeks into her first pregnancy.

Unbelievably, her world turned upside down again. Samantha was diagnosed with acute lymphocytic leukemia (ALL), a rapidly progressing cancer involving the blood and bone marrow that creates immature blood cells. "The leukemia had nothing to do with my previous diagnosis and treatment of breast cancer. It just happened to be a very rare, random cancer occurrence."

Heartbreakingly, Samantha's life became more of a struggle, with routines that dominated her life for many months: light doses of chemotherapy that would not affect her unborn child, and full quarantine in a hospital room because she was so immunocompromised that the smallest infection could kill her.

"I kept my sanity by taking long walks around the hospital floors, doing arm workouts with water bottles, and feeding off the incredible unending support from my husband, family, and friends. These simple routines consumed my days and made me feel purposeful."

Her medical team decided it was time to induce her labor at thirty-six weeks because she was considered full-term and Samantha couldn't delay more aggressive treatment any longer. Thankfully and happily, her daughter was born healthy.

"We, again, thought this was the worst thing that we would ever have to endure. Once I finished treatment and was told that I was in remission, I fell into a horrendous, debilitating depression. We weren't sure if it was delayed postpartum depression, post-traumatic stress disorder (PTSD), or a combination of the two, but it was the worst thing that I had ever experienced in my life. I wanted to die. For about three months, I spent every second of every day fighting off thoughts of suicide. My daughter was about six months old, and the only thing that kept me alive. She was my life, and she needed me."

Samantha was prescribed antidepressants, but they did nothing. She focused on her mindset instead. What did help was to concentrate on stopping the horrible, exhausting thoughts long enough to get her brain functioning enough to take the next steps.

"I started getting outside more; went on lots of walks with my husband, mom, and friends; and rode my stationary bike. I began eating nutritious foods again, and I started to feel a little better. I returned to work and finally started to feel more and more like me."

One of her close friends encouraged her to check out the Naples, Florida, Burn Boot Camp, and she did. Samantha began attending camp daily, and after a few weeks she finally felt like herself again.

"I loved the physical aspect, but even more than that, I loved the group of women and trainers that I got to see every day. I felt like I was part of a team again, and they reminded me of the second family I had as an athlete. After six months or so, I was in the best shape of my life. I had never felt stronger, more confident, nor more mentally tough."

But then came more catastrophic news: a third cancer diagnosis. It was discovered after her knee started bothering her. Samantha was diagnosed with osteosarcoma, also known as bone cancer, again unrelated to the prior cancers.

"The doctor could see that I was in shock, but fortunately it was curable. I would need very intense chemotherapy, along with major surgery to remove the bone tumor and later to rebuild my leg, and then back to chemo. Although I was grateful to be alive and to have my leg (formerly, amputation was the main treatment for this cancer), the mental and physical battle that I faced was beyond grueling. About two weeks after surgery, I resumed chemo."

How in the world can one maintain optimism or sanity as things keep getting worse?

Samantha concentrated on her mindset. "I knew I had to stay positive. Many people who beat cancer generally have a *positive attitude*. I knew that if I set my mind to just keeping my body moving, and I worked out at home, it would help. I was not exactly doing box jumps, but I could do other things, continue my mini-band work, and go on slow walks throughout the hospital corridors. Whenever there was an exercise I couldn't do, I would substitute it for a physical therapy exercise."

Samantha set her sights on hitting her 250th camp—an accomplishment she achieved on December 31, 2022.

"As I walked in that day, there were all the trainers, the full Burn staff, and even my Burn 'sisters.' I just figured everyone was there to end the year strong. But I realized that they had all shown up for me! They showered me with hugs, gifts, praise, and love. It was the best camp ever! I know that I would not have made it without each and every one of them."

No one has determined a perfect formula for helping cancer patients heal. Regardless, Samantha is convinced that a regular workout routine, with a group of supportive friends, makes a difference. When you connect with people who are good for you, you feel it, right down to your very being. She says: "Any activity that can shore up your support network— do it!"

We all know that a balanced diet and exercise program are important parts of becoming—and staying—healthy. But as we've noted, a growing body of evidence is showing that there is another factor that's as important for keeping our inner and outer strength strong: social connections.

Research tells us that our connections and the quality of those connections are bigger predictors of early death than obesity and physical activity and on par with smoking and excess alcohol consumption. Of course, it isn't just our physical health that suffers from a lack of connection; other studies show that having healthy romantic relationships also leads to better mental health, including less depression, and even helps ease the symptoms of severe stress. Without strong relationships or a close-knit group of friends, there's no psychological safety net. We should all be thinking as much about our relationships as we do about all other aspects of our health and well-being.

So—how can you enrich those relationships, build new ones, and enjoy the physical and mental health benefits of social connection?

CONNECT TO YOUR CORE IDENTITY FIRST.

True connection starts as an inside job. What happens after that, with effort and commitment, takes it over the line. A whole, balanced person is connected to their "core identity" and has an intrinsically connective spirit. So let's elaborate.

People have two identities: a surface identity and a core identity. When we first meet someone, they usually say something like "Hi, I'm Susan. I'm a banker at First National." They introduce themselves at only a fairly shallow level. This is their surface identity.

Surface identify is like the papery skin covering an onion. It doesn't go any deeper. If you're asked the question "Who are you?" you probably give a similar response—one that includes your name and what you do for a living. Yes, these answers explain parts of you, but they barely scratch the surface of who you are on the inside.

When we introduce ourselves, we don't say, "We're Devan and Morgan, CEOs of Burn Boot Camp." We introduce ourselves with our core identities: "We're married to each other, we're parents of three kids, and we're entrepreneurs. We're driven by our family and positively affecting every life we touch."

Who you really are is your core identity. It is like the interior of that onion, with many different layers—the multilayers of your being—involving your innermost needs and feelings. Who you are at your core affects how you bounce back from setbacks, interrelate with others, make decisions, and navigate life challenges. In short, it describes your overall psychological well-being.

You describe your core identity by knowing:

- Your strengths—what you're good at, the qualities that make you great, give you energy, and make you unforgettable

- Your purpose in life
- Your values—what you stand for (and against)
- Your style—not your taste in music, clothes, or interests, but rather knowing yourself well enough to know what you like, want, and need from life

Without knowing your core identity, it can be tough to navigate life. So it's important to dig deep and identify yourself at your core—what you truly care about in life. You don't do what society expects you to do, but what you want to do. You focus on what you care about.

In a nutshell, there are several benefits to connecting to your core identity:

Happiness. When you know yourself, understand yourself, and accept yourself, then you'll experience happiness—and what you really want to accomplish.

Clearer decision-making. For the most part, you are who you are today because of the choices you made yesterday. So, naturally, you'll want to make the best decisions you can. The more you know yourself, the clearer that process becomes, and you're more likely to make better choices about everything.

Self-control. One of the biggest strengths you can display is self-control. The ability to develop self-control depends on understanding yourself and what drives you. Self-control allows you to resist bad habits and develop good ones.

Better understanding of others. A hallmark of emotional intelligence is empathy—for yourself and for others. When you understand your own strengths and weaknesses better, you become a more empathetic and compassionate person and see things from another person's perspective. This ability is a superpower that can change lives.

Personal energy. Knowing who you truly are enriches your life and it is more exciting—which becomes contagious to those around you and strengthens your connection to them.

FRIENDSHIP AND COMMUNITY ARE VITAL.

From the time you were a little kid up through adulthood, chances are you've based a lot of your self-esteem on how many friends you have. It's just human nature to think the more friends you have the better. But is that true? And just how large should your friendship circle be?

The answer to this question comes from Robin Dunbar, an anthropologist and professor of evolutionary research at the University of Oxford. He has conducted extensive research on the matter and says the magic number is 150. If that sounds like a lot, he's talking about social connections rather than deep, meaningful friendships.

As Dunbar writes in the journal *Trends in Cognitive Sciences*, "Friendship is the single most important factor influencing our health, well-being, and happiness. Creating and maintaining friendships is, however, extremely costly, in terms of both the time that has to be invested and the cognitive mechanisms [the mental and emotional energy that goes into maintaining relationships] that underpin them."

He has concluded that our ability to handle social connections is limited to between 150 and 200, now referred to as "Dunbar's number." Interestingly, this number is rooted in history and evolution, and is about the size of the groups of our hunter-gatherer ancestors and the average Christmas card list.

But 150 is just part of the story. Dunbar theorized that the smallest and closest circle has just five people—loved ones. They are the ones who drive your passion and purpose in life.

This is followed by various layers of connection: 15 (good friends), 50 (friends), 150 (those meaningful connections), 500 (acquaintances), and 1,500 (people you can recognize). We float in and out of these layers, but the idea is that you're having to decide every day about how much time you want to invest in your social contacts, and that's limited. What matters most, however, is the quality of your friendships, not the quantity.

We recommend that you focus on nurturing those fifteen good friends, for starters. They should be real-life interactions, not virtual connections like Facebook "friends." Relationship experts note that the number of followers you have on social media has little, if any, impact on your well-being.

Write down who these fifteen people are. Then turn your mind for a moment to them and reflect on how much time you spend with them.

How often do you see those people or stay in touch with them? Daily? Monthly? Yearly? Do the math and estimate how many hours each year you spend with them.

Our social interactions play a role in our happiness. Scholars have found that, on average, "very happy" people socialize on eleven more occasions a year with loved ones than unhappy people do, seven more times with neighbors, and five more times with friends.

Of course, you don't have to spend every hour with your friends and loved ones. In fact, some relationships work better when there's some social distance. But if you have people in your life you'd like to see more often, ask yourself:

- Am I spending enough time with the people I care most about?
- Is there a relationship in my life that would benefit if both of us spent more time together?
- How can I nourish my relationships with friends and loved ones?
- Relationships require two people putting in the necessary effort. Who in my circle is willing to do that?

Take a few moments to draw up your current connections, then consider what you're receiving, what you're giving, and where you would like your relationships to go.

JOIN A FITNESS FACILITY OR GYM.

These days, fitness facilities are playing a larger role in fostering connections, enhancing wellness, and counteracting the more negative aspects of modern society, such as isolation due to technology and other factors. Not only do they provide group classes that build connections, but many are also being designed with lounge areas and other social spaces so that if you're between classes, you can drop into a café, healthy juice bar, or lounge and sit with friends in these social spaces. And where better to connect with people who share your goals than at a gym?

It's pretty easy to meet people in a gym or an exercise class, even if you're shy. Just start a conversation, like "These moves are challenging, right?" People will respond, and that's when you start talking more. Or you might compliment someone by noting how much progress they've made or how hard they work out.

Loneliness is responsible for more sickness, suffering, and death than almost anything else. When we find ourselves untethered, there's no substitute for authentic human connection. The reality is that we are increasingly separating from one another, and what we all need is people in our lives who really see us, hold us, and support who we're trying to become. To feel genuine belonging and acceptance helps us thrive. In sociology, it's called a "third place," home and work being first and second. It's a familiar environment where you are at your best. Where you regularly connect with others, known and unknown, over a shared interest or activity.

SEEK OUT CONNECTIONS AT A VARIETY OF OTHER PLACES AND EVENTS.

Insert yourself at events, venues, and other activities and surround yourself with new people. And don't be afraid to reach out first and initiate conversations. Some suggestions:

Volunteer for a Cause or Charity You Care About

You'll meet other people who are like-minded, all involved in an experience to bond over. The beneficial effects of volunteering on health have been well documented. It improves physical health, plus it helps you feel better mentally. It makes you feel more satisfied with your life, boosts your self-esteem, and brings greater happiness. It may even help extend your life.

Volunteering is a form of service, and service can be so many other things—little things. Letting someone get ahead of you in line or in traffic. Holding a door open. Lending a hand. Mentoring someone. Living a life full of kindness. And, of course, every aspect of parenting. There just needs to be a conscious intention and willingness to give the best you can, without expectations.

Network!

Joining business clubs or professional organizations is a great way to meet people who share similar business and professional interests. You get to know them, and vice versa. This is also a great way to build your business and enhance your professional life.

Check Out Facebook and Meetup Groups

Go on Facebook or Meetup.com and find groups in your area with similar interests: singles, gardening, book clubs, nutrition, outdoor sports, and more. It seems that Facebook and meetups have a group for anything and everything. Then start attending events organized for these groups. You'll share your favorite, common activities with other people—and tap into the potential for making long-lasting friendships.

Download a Friendship App

These apps are designed to help you find people who share your interests. You write your profile, list your interests and hobbies, and share your location—then almost instantly make connections. Whether you're a pet lover, a new parent, a sports fan, or a traveler, there is something for everyone.

Some friendship apps include: Bumble BFF (for meeting new friends), Nextdoor (for meeting nearby neighbors), Friender (for shared interests),

Skout (for people who like to travel or pursue certain hobbies), and Atleto (for athletes).

Use Your Friends to Make More

Tell your friends that you're doing a particular event or activity, ask whether they want to join—and bring some of their friends.

Make Friends with Other Parents

If you have kids, make friends with the parents of their classmates—the ones they like. You never know where the connection will lead. We've made a lot of friends through this avenue.

HANG AROUND WITH DOERS.

We're talking about positive, driven people who act on their goals—people who feel that if they can't do it, it can't be done! Really make an effort here. If you don't know people like this, find them and bring them into your circle.

Doers are the opposite of what we call "dabblers." A dabbler is someone who jumps around from gym to gym, from diet to diet, from job to job, and never really makes a commitment to lasting change. This person says they're going to commit to transforming their body for good—only to quit at the first sign of difficulty. They are super fired up when it's convenient but end up failing, pivoting in direction, and starting over at the first moment of demotivation.

But doers choose to do what's hard, and when they do that, their lives become easy, whereas dabblers choose to do what's easy, and their lives become hard.

The moral here: don't be a dabbler, be a doer. As you create your circle of connection, surround yourself with other doers. If you run into dabblers, it's okay to weed them out of your life. Dabblers can bring you down, and you need people in your circle of connection who will lift you up.

DEVELOP THE TRAITS OF HIGHLY CONNECTED PEOPLE.

Far too many people mistakenly believe that the ability to make friends is a natural trait possessed by only a lucky few. Not true! Being more sociable is completely doable and not that hard. It's a matter of developing your emotional intelligence and building just a few simple skills that will get you more connected. For example:

Leave a Great First Impression

Did you know that most people size you up within six to twelve seconds of meeting you, then decide whether they like you? This is fact, according to social psychologists, and backed by research. Sounds a little crazy, right? But knowing helps you create a better first impression.

How?

In one simple way: Be aware of your body language—your gestures, the way you carry yourself, your facial expressions, and your tone of voice. Be enthusiastic when you speak. Smile. Uncross your arms. Maintain eye contact. Lean in slightly to listen to the other person. These are all forms of positive body language that will draw people to you like ants at a picnic.

Be Interested in Others

It's tough to build relationships when you ask the same old questions, like "What do you do?" or "Where are you from?" or "How are you?" If you want to become interesting, first you must be genuinely interested. Meaning, being curious about other people is the best way for them to enjoy your company.

Honestly, the above questions make for shallow small talk. Instead, find out what makes the other person tick (without becoming too personal) and ask substantial questions, such as:

- Why did you choose your profession?
- What do you like about where you live?
- What activities do you enjoy?

- What's your family like?
- If you could travel anywhere in the world, where would you go?

Smile!

For millennia, the smile has been recognized as a powerful communication device. According to a 2019 review in *Postgraduate Medical Journal*, smiling is a sign of compassion, empathy, and friendliness. It also builds trust in relationships.

People gravitate to people who smile. If you want to attract new connections and get people to like you, smile during conversations. They will automatically feel good about you.

Look for Mutual Areas of Bonding

Your next great friendship usually won't come knocking on your door. You've got to get out there and put forth some effort, specifically toward people with whom you have something in common.

You're more likely to connect with someone over shared goals, a similar history, or mutual interests, even if you are complete strangers! If you meet someone who talks about wanting to get in better shape, for example, invite them to a fitness event, such as going to the gym, training for a 5K race, or attending a yoga class. Shared interests bring people closer together and forge stronger relationships.

Be an Active Listener

Being a great listener is a master skill for connection. It telegraphs that you're interested in a closer relationship.

A lot of conversations, however, tend to be just alternating monologues. No one is really listening, but rather thinking of what to say next while the other person is talking.

Too often, we underestimate the power of a listening ear, which has the potential to build connections, even turn a life around. Plus, when you listen, you learn more. But if someone opens up to you or shares something personal and you aren't actively listening, that person may not feel comfortable hanging out with you again.

Active listeners, on the other hand:

- Maintain eye contact
- Let the talker finish their story, thoughts, and communication
- Do not interrupt
- Use the person's name in conversation
- Ask follow-up questions about what they just heard
- Pay attention to areas of common interests or passions
- Use positive body language while listening, such as nods and smiles
- Put their phones out of sight
- Are not judgmental

Share Information About Yourself

It's okay to be vulnerable. Share yourself with others—your dreams, your hurts, your challenges. Doing so creates deep connection and gives other people a chance to really know you. Although this may feel scary and uncomfortable, research shows that self-disclosure makes you more likable.

Here's an analogy: Let's say you walk up to a restaurant. The lights are off, and there's a CLOSED sign on the door. You probably wouldn't go in, right?

Well, the same goes for people. If you're closed off and the other person senses it, you won't get very far with that connection.

But when you're willing to share personal things—your childhood, your dreams and goals, and challenges in life—it's like flipping on the light switch and hanging an OPEN sign on the door.

Check In from Time to Time

Friendship is like a garden full of flowers and plants, and the constant work you need to do to maintain a strong ongoing friendship is a bit like being a gardener. A gardener needs to tend to the flowers and plants regularly to make sure they're getting enough water and nutrients. The same is true when it comes to keeping important relationships alive.

So make it a habit to check in on your friends and loved ones to make sure they're okay. This isn't hard, nor is it time-consuming.

Consider doing one or more of the following:

- Make a weekly "catch-up" phone call
- Send an occasional text message to see how they're doing
- Send them an article about something they're interested in
- Invite them to events or to just hang out
- Send cards on special occasions

Genuinely Compliment People and Express Appreciation

We all want to feel admired and appreciated. It's just human nature. So give genuine compliments to people. Watch them bloom under your appreciation. When you make others happy, you'll feel happy too.

Our favorites:

- I love the way you push yourself in this exercise class. You're such an inspiration.
- You look great since you started your fitness program.
- You're a terrific cook. I tell everyone about the delicious dishes you prepare.
- Your positive attitude is so contagious and encouraging.
- I admire your persistence and determination.
- Thank you for making my life more wonderful.

You'll easily lift someone's spirits and draw them to you by acknowledging their work, attitude, style, accomplishments, appearance, or anything else you find commendable.

Sure, it's true people just "click," and there is such a thing as chemistry. But most of the time, it takes a certain amount of energy to build lasting connections. Remember that we're wired to connect with one another. And when we do, everyone wins—in terms of happiness, joy, and long-term well-being.

THE FINISHER

WE'VE COME TO THE END OF THE BOOK, AND WE'VE COVERED A LOT OF ground, but for you, this is really the beginning. We hope we have opened your eyes to the importance of achieving success and happiness in all areas of your life. More than that, though, we want you to know that you have everything within you to be truly healthy, successful, and happy. You are unique—there's no one like you on the entire planet. You have talents, insights, and value, all waiting to be tapped. You possess the potential to enjoy your life, your career, and your relationships. You're loved and you can love. You can gain control of things you thought were out of your control. You have the ability to accomplish big things. You are on a trajectory toward a great life. You just need clarity, consistency, and confidence to reestablish your power and momentum.

The time has come. No more making excuses or talking about it— that's easy. Doing it consistently is the challenge, and challenge is what creates character.

As you move forward in your life, never forget that our program boils down to five important strategies. Review them over and over to stay the course. As a handy refresher, here you go:

Burn. Start by moving your body in demanding, challenging ways. A body in motion stays in motion—in all things. A body stays at rest—also in all things. You must set yourself in motion. Moving changes your inner and outer strength so that you're more compelled and motivated to take action in other parts of your life. Make physical movement a priority, and the rest flows from there.

Believe. Change your attitude, self-talk, belief system, and level of effort. When these change for the better, everything in your life changes. Figure out what your unmet needs are. Once you identify them, you can meet those needs and move your life forward.

Nourish. Establish in your mind that food is fuel, and it is for the nourishment of your body and mind. Understanding and living this point is extremely powerful from here on out. Once you've cemented this mindset, the rest is easy. You'll start making food decisions that honor your body, shower it with self-love, and ditch the diet mentality that has kept you imprisoned for too much of your life.

Achieve. You might be coming from a bad place right now. It doesn't matter. What matters is where you're going. That new direction starts today with North Star goal-setting and taking small steps to achieve those goals. Tomorrow doesn't get better by wishing; it gets better by planning. And to plan, you need goals.

Connect. One of the most exciting findings in health research today is the power of social connections—friends and loved ones. We need them as much as we need nutritious food and daily physical activity. The making and nurturing of our close connections takes the friction out of life, provides a dose of joy, and makes our lives complete.

With these five strategies in mind, know exactly what you desire in the eight key areas of your life—body, mind, emotions, spirit, relationships, time, work, and money—and be on a clear path to transform them. By clarifying your North Star goals and devising a solid plan of action, by focusing, acquiring a positive attitude, putting forth effort, and connecting, a transformation will take place. You will change on the inside; therefore, your life will change. Hoped-for opportunities will come your way. Uplifting and encouraging people will be drawn to you. Your life will be headed in the wonderful direction you've always desired.

We challenge you to embrace the five strategies we've put forth, then implement them in your life. Every single day, you make choices that affect how you live, how happy you are, and what the future brings. Will you be healthy? Will you be fulfilled? Will you live with purpose? You're always one decision away from transforming your life. So choose very carefully!

Right now, you may not know what your next step is. That's okay; it often takes some energy to find your footing before venturing forward. What we suggest is that you write a letter to one of your closest friends, detailing what your goals are, what you want to do in your life, and what you'd like to transform over the next three to five years. This directs your effort, actions, and decisions toward whatever means the most to you.

Keep your letter simple and clear. Don't worry about length. Your letter should express how you expect to transform your life. Be positive. For example, don't write what you don't want to do or be. Rather, write what you want to do or become. Include positive behaviors, character qualities, and healthy habits that you want to develop further. Make it sound compelling, inspiring, and energizing.

Pick one to three North Star goals in each of the eight areas of life. Express to your friend the following: why you chose this goal, what the goal is, how you plan to accomplish the goal, and by when.

Mail it to your friend, but keep a copy handy. Refer to it often to gauge whether you're on track. Review it with your friend after six months.

If you need help getting started, here are some trigger phrases you can adapt:

- I will . . . [what you want to accomplish—your goals] . . . so that . . . [the reasons why these goals are important to you]. I will establish . . . [small steps you will take to get there].
- I will build a routine around the eight key areas of my life [by adapting key strategies].
- I will do . . . [choose actions you will do every day to advance your transformation].

- I will change . . . [choose attitudes, beliefs, and self-talk] . . . because . . . [reasons that making these changes are important to you].
- I am grateful for . . . [most important things to you].
- I want to be viewed as a person who is . . . [positive traits you want to develop].

You have not been alone in this journey. Everything we've shared with you comes from our hearts. We care about you; we care about your life. We're all about helping you change—the how and why to do it—and especially how you can move forward in your life. Now it's up to you. Your part is now most of it, and you are what will make it happen.

Whether you know what your next step is or not, use these true stories as inspiration to move forward toward a new level in your life. Just like Brian, who started his own Burn Boot Camp to help others the way it helped him. Just like Hope, who committed herself to her workouts to escape addiction. *You, too,* can have a story that embodies hope for the future, joy for living in the present, and freedom from a negative past.

At one time or another, we will all be faced with the decision to leap high walls—to do hard things and live life on our terms—to radically transform our lives. From this book, we hope you've drawn the guidance to make that happen.

So now the real journey begins. And the destination? A long, healthy, and purpose-filled life where you get to enjoy what you love, with who you love, where you love, all while feeling energetic and enthusiastic for life!

APPENDIX A
THE BURN BOOT CAMP
BODYWEIGHT EXERCISES

Jumping Jacks

Target: Abdominals, shoulders, glutes, calves, hamstrings, and quadriceps. This exercise also elevates your heart rate for a conditioning benefit.

Start: Position your feet about hip width apart, evenly distribute your weight, and keep your knees bent slightly. Stay tall with a neutral head and neck position. Keep your arms by your sides.

Action: Jump your feet outside your hips, while raising your arms overhead. Jump back to the starting position, lowering your arms back down.

Repeat for the recommended time or number of repetitions.

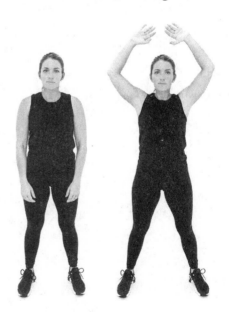

Reverse Crunches

Target: Abdominals, core

Start: Lie on your back on the floor or an exercise mat. Place your hands palms down at your sides.

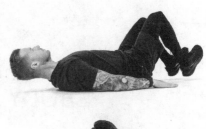

Action: Bend your knees slightly and bring them toward your head, drawing them upward toward the end of the move. Slowly return to the starting position.

Repeat for the recommended time or number of repetitions.

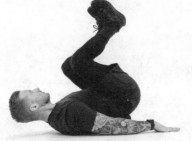

Mountain Climbers

Target: Abdominals, lower back, hamstrings, and glutes. Mountain climbers help raise your heart rate, but are also a low-impact exercise, which is easy on your joints.

Start: Start in the traditional push-up position. Your spine and legs should all form a straight line, with your elbows locked and your hands placed directly beneath your shoulders. Keep your core engaged.

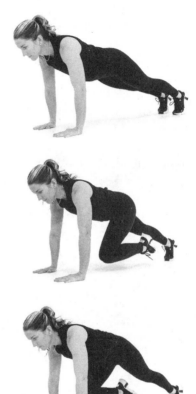

Action: Bring your left knee into your chest and place your left foot on the floor. Straighten your left leg and jump it to the starting position, while simultaneously pulling your right leg up toward your chest.

Alternate this motion at a fast pace for the recommended time length or number of repetitions. This exercise should be done as if you are running in place from the push-up position.

Power Planks

Target: Abdominals, hips, lower back, and shoulders

Start: Get into a high plank position. Then prop yourself up on your forearms, shoulder width apart. Lift your body up so that you are also propped up by your toes. Hold your hands together, with your palms flat on the floor, or position your hands so your palms are facing each other with your thumbs up.

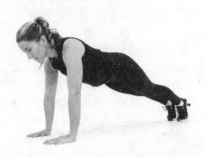

Action: Draw in your navel toward your spine, squeeze your glutes, tuck your tailbone under, and slightly squeeze the bottom points of your shoulder blades. Hold this position for the recommended amount of time.

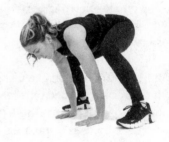

High Knee Sprinters

Target: Quadriceps, hamstrings, calves, glutes, and hip flexors. This exercise also improves conditioning fitness, muscular endurance, balance, and coordination.

Start: Stand tall and position your feet about shoulder width apart. Hold your arms at your sides. Tighten your core muscles.

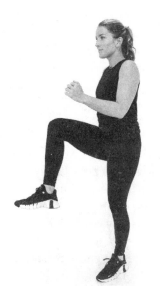

Action: Bend your right knee and lift it up toward your chest, slightly above waist level. Simultaneously, move your left arm up, elbow bent, in a pumping motion.

Quickly lower your right knee and left arm. Repeat with your left knee and right arm. Alternate your right and left knees (and arms) for the recommended time.

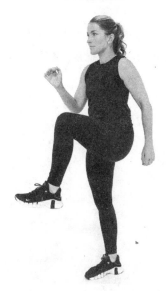

Half Burpees

Target: Hamstrings, glutes, triceps, abdominals, deltoids, quadriceps, lower back, and calf muscles. Half burpees also improve conditioning fitness.

Start: Stand with your feet together. Flex your knees and put your palms on the floor in front of your feet, slightly wider than your shoulders.

Action: Kick both feet out behind you so that you are in a high plank position. All in one motion jump your big toes to your pinky fingers while palms remain flat on the floor. Lift palms off the floor and jump with hands over head. Continue to kick your feet back and forth in a controlled manner for the recommended number of repetitions.

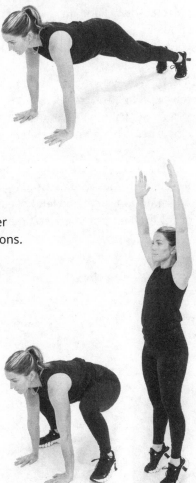

Full Burpees

Target: Legs, hips, buttocks, abdomen, arms, chest, and shoulders—and of course, conditioning fitness

Start: Stand with your feet together. Flex your knees and put your palms on the floor in front of your feet, slightly wider than your shoulders.

Action: Kick both feet out behind you so that you are in a high plank position. Keep your core engaged and your spine straight. Perform a push-up.

After you finish the push-up, jump your feet up toward your chest and land in a squat position.

Jump in the air with your arms above your head. Land and repeat the exercise for the recommended number of reps.

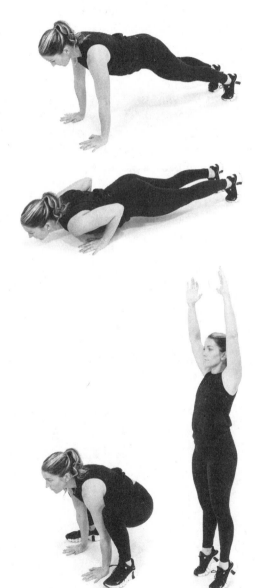

Shoulder Taps

Target: Abdominals, back, chest, arms, muscular endurance, and stability

Start: Position your body in a high plank, with your feet about hip width apart. Square your hips and shoulders, and maintain a neutral spine.

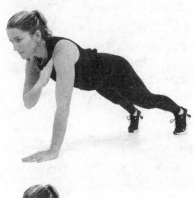

Action: Lift up your right hand, and tap your left shoulder. Place your right hand back on the floor. Lift up your left hand to tap your right shoulder, then put it back on the floor.

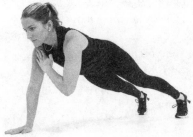

Repeat for the recommended time length or number of repetitions.

Renegade Rows

Target: Back and core

Start: Get in a high plank position. Keep your back flat. Spread your feet a little wider than shoulder width.

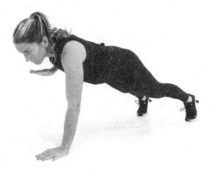

Action: Perform a full push-up. After the push-up, bend your right elbow, and "row" up, contracting your lateral muscle at the top of the move. Do not rotate your hips. Lower your right arm back to the floor and repeat on the left side. That's one complete rep.

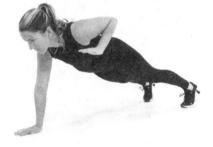

Repeat for the desired time length or number of repetitions.

Note: You have the option to use dumbbells to perform the rowing motion.

Thoracic Rotations

Target: Core, plus middle and upper back. This exercise also improves your upper-back mobility and posture.

Start: Position yourself on your hands and knees, with your hands directly beneath your shoulders.

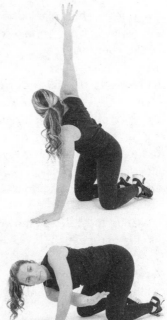

Action: Rotate your right arm, head, and upper back toward the ceiling as far as you can. Next, reach under and across your body while your opposite arm remains straight. Return to the starting position, and repeat the same motion but on the left side.

Alternate from right to left for the desired time length or recommended number of repetitions.

Rapid-Fire Punches

Target: Shoulders, biceps, core, and triceps

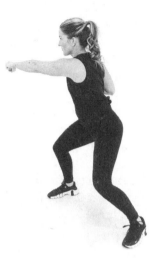

Start: Stand tall and place your feet about shoulder width apart. Keep your core engaged. Bend your elbows and raise your fists up in front of your face as boxers do.

Action: Transfer your weight to your right foot. Pivot on your left foot, and rotate your trunk toward the right as you throw your left punch across your body.

Return to the starting position, and repeat the motion on your opposite side. Keep your core tight throughout the move.

Continue for 30 seconds as fast as you can, and then rest for 30 seconds.

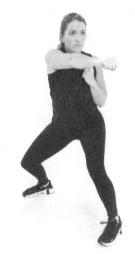

Arm Circles

Target: Shoulders, rotator cuffs, and upper arms

Start: Stand tall and place your feet about shoulder width apart. Extend your arms out to both sides of your body, at shoulder height.

Action: Make large circles (about a foot in diameter). Go forward for about 10 seconds, then backward for 10 seconds.

Repeat the motion for the desired time length or recommended number of repetitions.

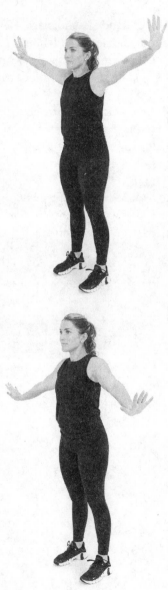

Heismans

Target: Legs, core, hips, glutes; strength, speed, agility, and conditioning fitness

Start: Stand tall and place your feet about shoulder width apart. Bend your knees slightly and keep your arms at your sides.

Action: Hop off your left foot, take two small shuffle steps laterally, and land on your right foot, lifting your inside knee and pumping your right arm forward.

Immediately hop to your left, reversing the motion of your arms and legs.

Continue alternating from side to side. Don't let both feet touch the floor at the same time.

Repeat for the desired time length or recommended number of repetitions.

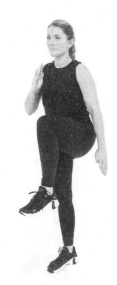

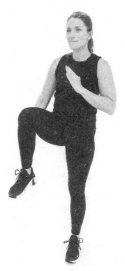

Dot Drill

Target: Balance, coordination, agility, leg strength, ankle and knee stability, and conditioning fitness

Start: Stand tall with your arms at your sides and your feet shoulder width apart.

Action: Move in-in, out-out on the balls of your feet, one foot at a time, with as much speed as possible. Pretend there are four dots on the floor. Two under your feet in starting position and two more dots 1–2 feet (one on each side) to the outside. Step on these dots with speed and accuracy.

Repeat this sequence for the desired time length or number of repetitions.

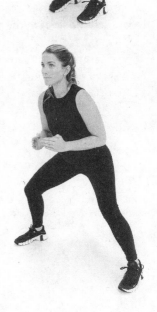

Skater Hops

Target: Glutes, quadriceps, and calves, while also improving balance and coordination

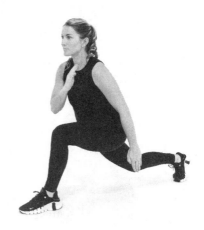

Start: This is a plyometric exercise that involves jumping from side to side, mimicking the movement of a skater on ice. Stand tall and place your feet shoulder width apart. Keep your arms at your sides.

Action: Shift your weight onto your left foot and lift your right foot off the floor. Push off laterally 1–2 feet. Bend your left knee, hop to the right, and land on your right foot.

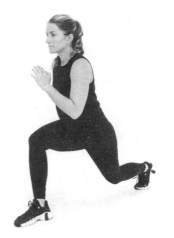

Immediately shift your weight onto your right foot and lift your left foot off the floor. Bend your right knee, hop to the left, and land on your left foot.

Continue hopping back and forth for the desired number of repetitions or time.

Bear Crawls

Target: Core, back, arms, and legs

Start: Start this exercise in a "bear" position. Place your hands on the floor a few feet in front of you, with your palms beneath your shoulders, knees bent and directly under your hips. Keep your core engaged.

Action: Start crawling on your hands and feet. Don't let your knees touch the floor.

Keep crawling forward for the recommended number of steps or distance.

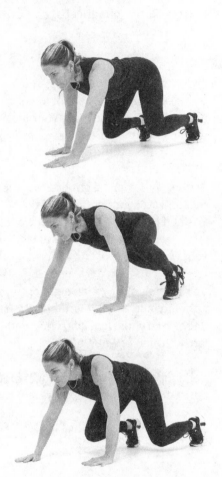

Chair Step-Ups

Target: Quadriceps, hamstrings, and glutes

Start: You'll need a sturdy chair or other sturdy elevated surface. Place your left foot on the chair.

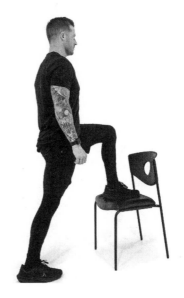

Action: Shift your weight into your right foot to step up onto the chair with your left foot. Bring your right knee to your chest and then return to start. If balance is an issue, simply bring your right foot to a standing position on the chair to increase stability.

Repeat for the desired time length or recommended number of repetitions.

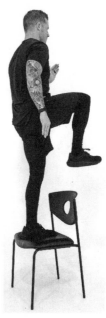

Hamstring Scoops

Target: Hamstrings, glutes

Start: Stand tall and place your feet about shoulder width apart.

Action: Place your left foot in front of the other with your left heel on the floor. Point your toes up.

Lower your body. Sit back on your butt while reaching your hands down, "scooping" the floor. The lower you sit, the more you'll feel it in your hamstrings. Hold for 2 to 3 seconds each time. Then stand back up.

Repeat the motion on the opposite side.

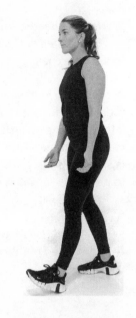

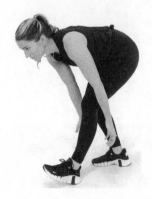

Low Runner Lunges

Target: Glutes, hips, and thighs

Start: Start by lunging left leg forward at a 90-degree angle and extend the right leg backward.

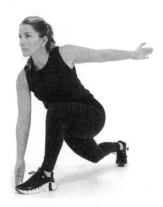

Action: Try to sink as low as you can, keeping your core engaged. Hold the posture, keeping your chest up and square to the wall in front of you.

Repeat on the other side, and alternate legs (and arms).

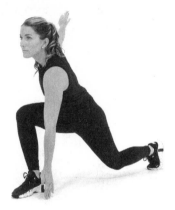

Butt Kickers

Target: Hamstrings, quadriceps, calves, and conditioning fitness

Start: Stand tall and place your feet about shoulder width apart. Keep your arms at your sides. Bend your knees slightly.

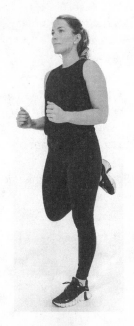

Action: Flex your right knee and lift it up to about waist level. Let your right foot kick your right glute. Return your right foot to the floor.

Then flex your left knee. Bring your left foot up behind you so that your heel kicks your left glute.

Alternate your kicks. Increase your speed until you're practically jogging in place.

Continue for the recommended time.

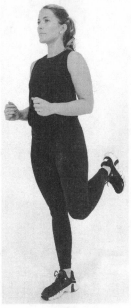

Squats

Target: Quadriceps, hamstrings, and glutes

Start: Stand tall and place your feet about hip width apart. Point your toes slightly outward. Keep your chest upright. Cross your arms over your chest or extend them out in front of your chest (elbows bent). Keep your eyes forward and head up.

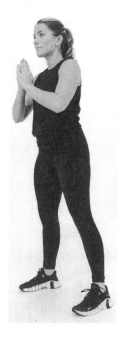

Action: Bend at the knees until your glutes are a couple inches above the floor. Lean your torso forward slightly as you go down, until your shoulders are just slightly over your knees. Slowly stand back up, returning to the starting position.

Repeat the squat for the recommended number of repetitions.

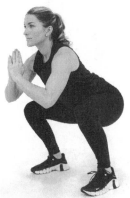

Sumo Squats

Target: Quadriceps, interior thighs, hamstrings, and glutes

Start: Stand tall, with your feet slightly wider than hip width and your toes pointed outward. Keep your back straight and hold your arms out in front of you, with elbows bent.

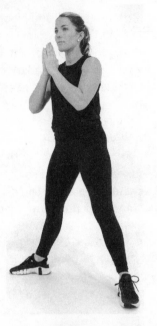

Action: Drop your hips until your thighs are parallel to the floor. Keep your core tight, back straight, and knees forward.

Push back up to the starting position, squeezing your glutes tightly at the top.

Repeat the squat for the recommended number of repetitions.

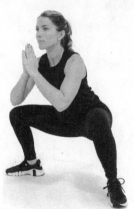

Reverse Lunges

Target: Quadriceps, hamstrings, glutes

Start: Stand tall and place your feet about shoulder width apart, toes pointed straight ahead. Engage your core.

Action: Take a large step backward as far as you can with your left foot. Flex your knees and lower your hips so that your right thigh is parallel to the floor. This is one lunge.

Push yourself back up with your left foot, and step forward so that your feet are together again. Repeat the motion on the opposite side.

Alternate left and right for the recommended number of repetitions.

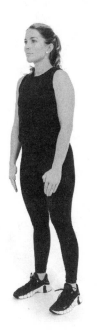

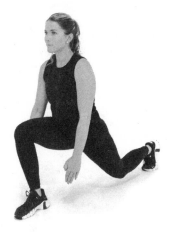

Forward Lunges

Target: Quadriceps, hamstrings, and glutes

Start: Stand tall and place your feet about shoulder width apart, toes pointed straight ahead. Engage your core.

Action: Step forward on your left foot, flexing your knees and lowering your hips until your left thigh is parallel to the floor. Your front knee should be over your toes but not past them. This is one lunge.

Step back to the starting position. Repeat the exercise for the recommended number of repetitions.

Repeat on the opposite leg.

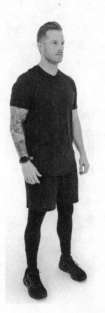

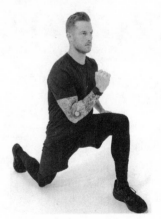

Alternating Lateral Lunges

Target: Quadriceps, inner thighs, and glutes

Start: Stand tall and place your feet about hip width apart, with your toes pointed forward.

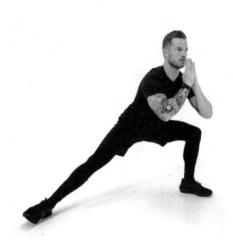

Action: Shift your weight onto your right foot. With your core engaged, lower your hips straight down. Your left leg should stay straight. Lower until your right thigh is nearly parallel to the floor.

Press into your right heel to return to the standing position.

Repeat the motion with your left leg, then again on the right leg, alternating legs throughout the exercise. This exercise basically works in a side-to-side motion.

Split Squats

Target: Quadriceps, hamstrings, and glutes

Start: Stand straight with your feet in a staggered stance. Your left foot should be forward and your right foot slightly back.

Action: Bend at both knees and lower yourself down till your left knee is parallel to the floor. Then stand back up.

Repeat this motion for the desired amount of repetitions. Then repeat the exercise on the opposite side.

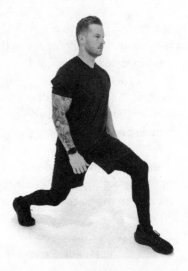

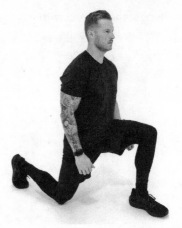

Wall Sit

Target: Quadriceps, hamstrings, and glutes

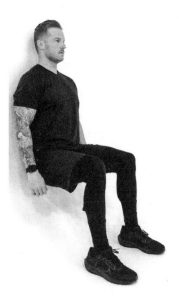

Start: Stand with your back and glutes against a wall. Next, walk your feet out away from the wall, and place them shoulder width apart and create a slight angle from your knees to your heels. Do not place your hands on your thighs; this makes the exercise less difficult.

Action: Bending at your knees, slowly lower your body until your thighs are parallel to the floor. Your knees should be directly above your feet and bent at a 90-degree angle.

Hold this position for the designated amount of time. Push yourself back up until your legs are straight again. Repeat.

Calf Raises

Target: Calf muscles

Start: Stand tall and place your feet about hip width apart. Point your toes forward. Flex your knees slightly and hold your hands by your sides or place them on your hips.

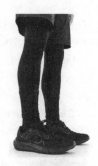

Action: Lift your heels up by pressing the balls of your feet into the floor until you are on your toes. Hold this position and then slowly lower your heels back to the floor.

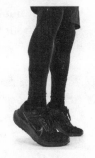

Repeat the exercise for the recommended number of repetitions. You can also perform this exercise on the edge of any stair or elevated stable platform.

Glute Bridges

Target: Glutes, hamstrings, and core

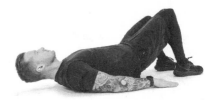

Start: Lie on your back on the floor. Position your feet about shoulder width apart, with your knees bent. Place your arms at your sides, with palms facing down.

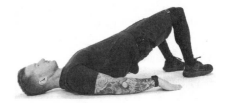

Action: Slowly lift your hips as high as you can. Tighten your glutes, and squeeze your abs at the top of the exercise. Hold this position for several seconds.

Slowly lower your hips back down to the floor, keeping the tension in your abs and glutes.

Repeat for the desired time length or recommended number of repetitions.

Single-Leg Glute Bridges

Target: Glutes, hamstrings, and core

Start: Lie on your back on the floor. Position your feet about shoulder width apart, with your knees bent. Place your arms at your sides, with palms facing down.

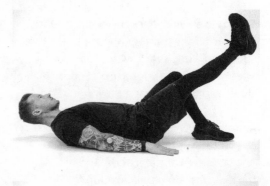

Action: Raise your hips up as high as you can, engaging your core and tightening your glutes.

Lift one leg upward, extending it fully so it is roughly 45 degrees to the floor.

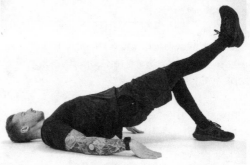

Hold this position for a count of one or two.

Lower the leg. Return to the starting position by lowering your hips to the floor.

Repeat on the same leg for the desired number of reps. Then switch legs.

Jump Squats

Target: Glutes, quadriceps, and hamstrings

Start: Stand tall and place your feet
shoulder width apart.

Action: Bend your knees and lower into
a full squat position until your thighs are
parallel to the floor. Propel your body up
and jump off the floor.

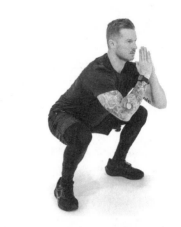

Then return to the start position.
Descend into the squat again for another
explosive jump.

Continue jump-squatting for the
recommended number of repetitions.

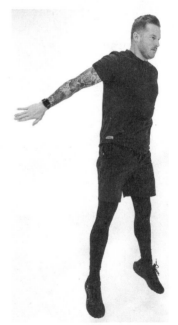

Jump Lunges

Target: Glutes, thighs, hamstrings, core, and calves. Not only is this an effective cardiovascular exercise, but it also develops stability and coordination.

Start: Step forward on your left leg into a lunge position. Lean slightly forward and tighten your core muscles.

Action: Jump upward, switching leg positions just before you land.

Once you land, drop to a deep lunge position. Start the next jump lunge on the opposite leg.

Repeat the movement, alternating legs.

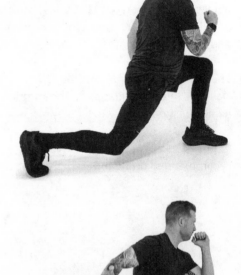

Walkouts

Target: Core and shoulders

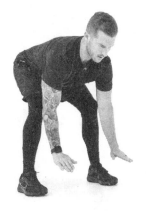

Start: Stand tall and place your feet about hip width apart. Bend your knees slightly. Hinge at your hips, reach for the floor, and place your palms in front of your feet.

Action: Shift your weight onto your hands and walk them forward until your body forms a straight line from your head to your heels (plank position). Tighten your core, and make sure your hands are directly under your shoulders.

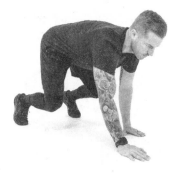

Walk back to the starting position and repeat the exercise for the recommended number of repetitions.

Push-Ups

Target: Shoulders, triceps, biceps, hip muscles, core, and the erector spinae muscle

Start: Start from a high plank position, with your hands directly below your shoulders. Keep your elbows slightly bent.

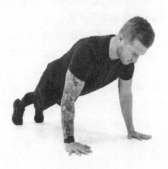

Action: Push yourself up off the floor. Keep your body in a straight line, with your core tight. Bend your elbows, and lower your chest to the floor. Ideally, touch your chest to the floor.

Push back up through your hands, returning to the starting position.

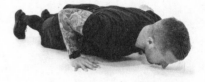

Repeat the exercise for the recommended number of repetitions.

Diamond Push-Ups

Target: Triceps, shoulders, biceps, hip muscles, core, and spinal muscles

Start: Start from a high plank position. Keep your elbows slightly bent.

In this variation, place your hands close together. Your thumb and index finger of one hand should touch those of the other hand, making a diamond shape on the floor.

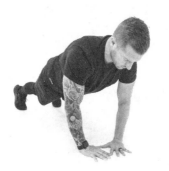

Action: Push yourself up off the floor. Keep your body in a straight line, with your core tight. Bend your elbows, and lower your chest to the floor.

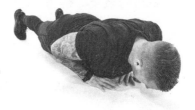

Push back up through your hands, returning to the starting position.

Repeat the exercise for the recommended number of repetitions.

Chair Tricep Dips

Target: Triceps

Start: Use a sturdy chair or bench. Place your hands about shoulder width apart, with your knuckles forward, on the edge of the chair. Extend your glutes slightly past the chair. In the upward position, place your body at a 90-degree angle with your feet flat on the floor.

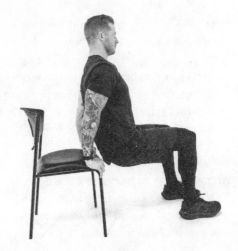

Action: To dip, lower yourself as far as possible. Your elbows should point behind you. Tighten your core, and squeeze your triceps on the way up.

Continue dipping down and pushing up for the recommended number of repetitions.

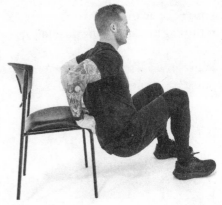

Plank-Ups

Target: Triceps, biceps, shoulders, abdominals, glutes, and hamstrings

Start: Place your body in a plank position, with your forearms on the floor or exercise mat. Your elbows should be directly underneath your shoulders, with your legs hip width apart. All repetitions should begin from this starting position. Keep your core engaged.

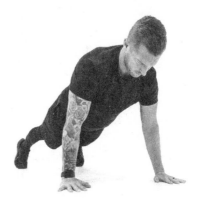

Action: Push up onto your hands, one arm at a time.

Then lower back down to your forearms, one forearm at a time.

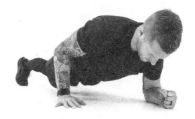

Continue to alternate between the forearm plank and push-up position for the recommended number of repetitions.

Supermans

Target: Back, core, hamstrings, and glutes

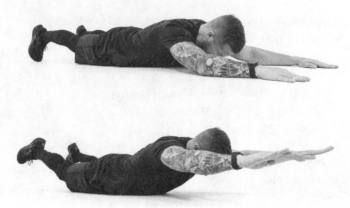

Start: Lie flat on your stomach. Extend your arms directly out in front of you. Keep your legs and arms straight.

Action: Simultaneously, lift your legs and arms off the floor as far as you can. Briefly pause at the top of the movement for 1 or 2 seconds—a position that looks as though you're flying like Superman.

Then slowly lower your arms and legs back to the starting position.

Repeat the exercise for the recommended number of repetitions.

Superman Lat Squeezes

Target: Back, core, hamstrings, and glutes

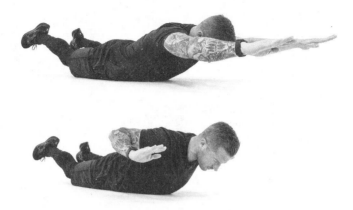

Start: Lie flat on your stomach. Extend your arms directly out in front of you. Keep your legs and arms straight.

Action: Simultaneously, lift your legs and arms off the floor as far as you can. Briefly pause at the top of the movement for 1 or 2 seconds—like Superman.

At this point, flex your elbows and pull your shoulder blades back as if you are performing a lateral pull-down. Squeeze your lats.

Then slowly return to the starting position.

Repeat the exercise for the recommended number of repetitions.

Low Plank Hold

Target: Abdominals, core, hips, lower back, and shoulders

Start: Begin in the low plank position. Your elbows should be aligned with your shoulders and your forearms out in front of you.

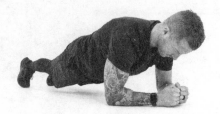

Action: Simply rest on your elbows and forearms as you hold the plank position.

Low Side Plank Hold

Target: Abdominals, core, glutes, hamstrings, and lower back muscles

Start: Prop your upper body with your forearm and elbow directly underneath your shoulder. With your legs extended, place one foot on top of the other.

Action: Lift your hips. Balance on your forearm and the side of your bottom foot.

Hold for the designated time. Switch sides and repeat.

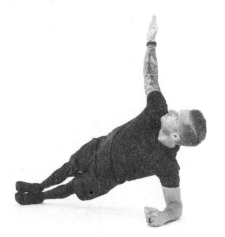

Scissor Kicks

Target: Abdominals, core, and hip flexors

Start: Lie on your back. Place your arms at your sides, palms down. Your lower back should be pressed into the floor.

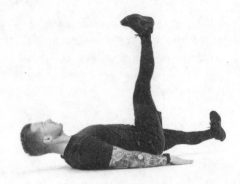

Action: Lift both legs about 6 inches off the floor, holding them at roughly a 45-degree angle, with your toes pointed.

Lift your right leg as high as you can; hold your left leg in space. Then lower your right leg to about 45 degrees while lifting your left leg as high as you can. That's one rep.

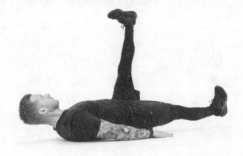

Continue alternating your legs in scissor fashion, while keeping them as straight as possible.

Bicycle Crunch

Target: Abs and core

Start: Lie down on your back with your legs straight and your hands behind your head. Tighten your core.

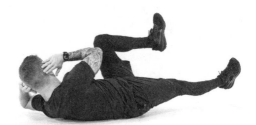

Action: Lift your shoulder blades off the floor. Lift your knees to about a 90-degree angle. Alternate extending your legs as if you're pedaling a bicycle. Rotate your body to touch your elbow to the opposite knee with each pedal motion.

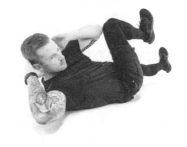

Flutter Kicks

Target: Core, abdominals, and quadriceps

Start: Lie on your back with your hands under your glutes and your head raised slightly above the floor. Keep your legs straight and together.

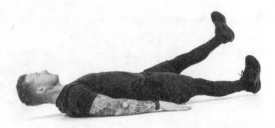

Action: Lift your legs 4 to 6 inches off the floor. Then lift one leg higher than the other. Bring it back down even with the other leg (which is still 4 to 6 inches off the floor). Repeat the motion with the opposite leg. Move in a swift, fluttering, up-and-down motion.

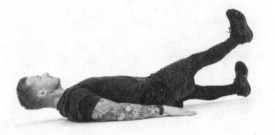

Repeat for the desired time length or recommended number of repetitions.

APPENDIX B
THE BURN 10-MINUTE MEAL PLAN RECIPES

* Recipes used in our meal plans

Unless otherwise indicated, the yield of each recipe is one serving.

BREAKFASTS

*Cinnamon Oat Muffin

Vegetable oil spray
¼ cup rolled oats
½ scoop Afterburn vanilla
   protein powder or other
   vanilla protein powder
1 teaspoon almond butter
¼ cup water
Ground cinnamon

Spray a single-serving muffin cup with vegetable oil. Preheat the oven to 350°F.

In a small bowl, combine all the ingredients, including cinnamon to taste, and mix well.

Pour into the prepared muffin cup. Bake for 12 minutes.

Nutrition: 164 calories, 15 grams protein, 17 grams carbohydrate, and 5 grams fat

Cinnamon Ezekiel French Toast

1 large egg
1 large egg white
¼ teaspoon ground cinnamon
¼ teaspoon pure vanilla
  extract
2 slices Ezekiel bread
Coconut oil spray
1 tablespoon pure maple
  syrup, for serving

In a small bowl, whisk together the egg, egg white, cinnamon, and vanilla. Soak the bread slices in the egg mixture. Spray a 10-inch skillet with the coconut oil, then cook the slices over medium heat until browned on both sides. Serve with maple syrup.

Nutrition: 302 calories, 14 grams protein, 49 grams carbohydrate, and 6 grams fat

*No-Bake Oats

⅓ cup rolled oats
1 scoop Afterburn vanilla
  protein powder or other
  vanilla protein powder
2 tablespoons powdered
  peanut butter
2 teaspoons ground flaxseed
⅓ cup unsweetened
  almond milk
½ banana, sliced
Pinch of ground cinnamon

In a small bowl, mix all the ingredients, except the banana and cinnamon. Refrigerate overnight. Then top with banana and cinnamon.

Nutrition: 300 calories, 24 grams protein, 40 grams carbohydrate, and 8 grams fat

Sweet Oats and Honey

½ cup rolled oats
½ scoop Afterburn vanilla
    protein powder or other
    vanilla protein powder
1 teaspoon honey
Pinch of ground cinnamon

Cook the oats according to the package directions. Stir in the protein powder, honey, and cinnamon.

Nutrition: 428 calories, 38 grams protein, 45 grams carbohydrate, and 10 grams fat

Avocado Protein Sandwich

2 slices Ezekiel bread
3 large egg whites, scrambled
2 slices pitted and peeled
    avocado
1 tablespoon feta cheese

Toast the bread. Top each slice with half the egg whites, an avocado slice, and half the cheese.

Nutrition: 275 calories, 21 grams protein, 33 grams carbohydrate, and 7 grams fat

Goat Cheese Omelet

Vegetable oil spray
1 cup egg whites, lightly
  beaten
1 well-packed cup spinach
1 ounce goat cheese

Spray a small skillet with vegetable oil. Heat the skillet over medium heat, add the egg whites and cook until lightly set.

Add the spinach, then the goat cheese. Continue to cook until the egg whites are set. Fold the omelet in half and serve.

Nutrition: 234 calories, 34 grams protein, 2 grams carbohydrate, and 9 grams fat

*Green Omelet with Ezekiel Bread

Vegetable oil spray
1 cup kale
1 cup egg whites, slightly
  beaten
2 slices Ezekiel raisin bread
1 tablespoon almond butter

Spray a small skillet with vegetable oil. Heat the skillet over medium heat, add the kale, and sauté until wilted. Remove from the heat and set aside.

Spray another small skillet with vegetable oil. Heat the skillet over medium heat, add the egg whites and cook until lightly set. Add the cooked kale over the egg whites. Continue to cook until the egg whites are set. Fold the omelet in half.

Serve with Ezekiel raisin bread, spread with the almond butter.

Nutrition: 428 calories, 38 grams protein, 45 grams carbohydrate, and 10 grams fat

Paleo Frittata

1 tablespoon olive oil
1 cup frozen mixed vegetables
½ cup liquid egg whites
1 large egg, beaten

In a small skillet, heat the olive oil over medium heat and sauté the vegetables until cooked throughout. Add the liquid egg whites and beaten egg. Continue to cook until the eggs are firm and set.

Nutrition: 224 calories, 20 grams protein, 12 grams carbohydrate, and 9 grams fat

Baked Eggs in Avocado

½ ripe avocado, pitted
1 large egg
Salt and freshly ground black pepper

Preheat the oven to 425°F.

Remove a few teaspoons of the avocado pulp to make room for the egg. Crack the egg into the opening created in the avocado half. Bake in a small baking dish for 15 minutes. Season to taste.

Nutrition: 233 calories, 8 grams protein, 9 grams carbohydrate, and 20 grams fat

Turkey and Veggie Casserole

Vegetable oil spray
4 ounces lean ground turkey
½ cup chopped mushrooms
¼ cup chopped onion
¼ cup seeded and chopped
   red bell pepper
½ cup egg whites

Preheat the oven to 425°F. Spray a small baking dish with vegetable oil.

Combine all the remaining ingredients in a small bowl. Mix well. Transfer the mixture to the prepared baking dish.

Bake for 40 to 45 minutes, or until set and cooked through.

Nutrition: 247 calories, 43 grams protein, 12 grams carbohydrate, and 2 grams fat

Afterburn Pancakes

Vegetable oil spray
¼ cup rolled oats
¼ cup plain fat-free Greek
   yogurt
½ scoop Afterburn vanilla
   protein powder or other
   vanilla protein powder
½ cup egg whites
Pinch of ground cinnamon,
   or ¼ teaspoon pure vanilla
   extract (optional)
Pure maple syrup, for serving
   (optional)

Spray a 10-inch skillet or griddle with vegetable oil.

Combine all the remaining ingredients in a small bowl and mix well. Heat the prepared pan over medium heat. Spoon the batter onto the skillet to form two or three small pancakes. Cook the pancakes on each side until lightly browned. Serve with maple syrup, if desired.

Nutrition: 229 calories, 33 grams protein, 18 grams carbohydrate, and 2 grams fat

*Greek Yogurt Parfait with Fruit

Drop of pure vanilla extract
Liquid stevia (optional)
⅔ cup plain fat-free yogurt
½ cup blackberries
½ cup strawberries
½ banana, sliced

Mix the vanilla and stevia (if using) into the yogurt. In a parfait glass, layer the yogurt alternately with the fruit.

Nutrition: 290 calories, 20 grams protein, 36 grams carbohydrate, and 4 grams fat

MAIN DISHES

Chicken Basil Spaghetti

1 raw medium-size spaghetti squash
Olive or avocado oil
Salt and freshly ground black pepper
2 ounces cooked chicken breast, cut into chunks
2 cherry tomatoes, halved
2 tablespoons chopped black olives
2 tablespoons cheese crumbles
1 tablespoon chopped fresh basil
Italian seasoning (optional)

Preheat the oven to 400°F.

Slice the spaghetti squash in half lengthwise, and scoop out the seeds. Drizzle with a little olive oil, and season to taste with salt and pepper. Place cut side down on a baking sheet. Bake until the squash can be easily shredded with a fork, about 40 minutes. Measure 1 cup of shredded squash for use in this recipe.

Layer the squash, chicken, tomatoes, olives, and cheese on a plate. Top with basil, Italian seasoning (if using), and more olive oil.

Nutrition: 277 calories, 22 grams protein, 14 grams carbohydrate, and 15 grams fat

Chicken and Cauliflower "Fried Rice"

Vegetable oil spray
¼ cauliflower head
1 cup chopped broccoli
¼ cup chopped onion
1 large egg, beaten
4 ounces cooked chicken
2 tablespoons coconut aminos

Spray a 10-inch skillet with vegetable oil. Pulse the cauliflower in a food processor until it forms a "rice" consistency. In the prepared skillet, combine the riced cauliflower, broccoli, and onion. Sauté over medium heat until soft. Add the egg and cook until set, stirring well. Add the chicken and coconut aminos. Heat throughout and serve.

Nutrition: 332 calories, 40 grams protein, 23 grams carbohydrate, and 9 grams fat

*Classic Chicken and Sweet Potato Meal

6 ounces cooked chicken
1 (4-ounce) baked sweet
   potato
1 cup steamed brussels
   sprouts

Plate all the ingredients for a quick nutritious meal.

Nutrition: 359 calories, 48 grams protein, 33 grams carbohydrate, and 5 grams fat

*Lean Spaghetti and Meatballs

1 medium-size spaghetti
  squash
Olive or avocado oil
Salt and freshly ground black
  pepper
4 ready-to-cook prepared
  meatballs
¼ cup marinara sauce

Preheat the oven to 400°F.

Slice the spaghetti squash in half lengthwise, and scoop out the seeds. Drizzle with a little olive oil, and season to taste with salt and pepper. Place cut side down on a baking sheet and bake until the squash can be shredded with a fork, about 40 minutes. Measure 1 cup of shredded squash for use in this recipe.

In a small skillet over medium heat, brown the meatballs until cooked through. Add the marinara sauce. Toss well.

Serve the meatballs and marinara over the squash.

Nutrition: 360 calories, 34 grams protein, 18 grams carbohydrate, and 17 grams fat

Grilled Chicken Parm and Zucchini Pasta

Vegetable oil spray
1 medium-size zucchini,
  spiralized
½ cup cherry tomatoes
1 garlic clove, minced
4 ounces grilled chicken
1 tablespoon grated Romano
  cheese

Spray a small skillet with vegetable oil, then add the zucchini, tomatoes, and garlic. Sauté over medium heat until the vegetables are soft. Transfer to a plate. Top with the chicken and cheese.

Nutrition: 220 calories, 33 grams protein, 9 grams carbohydrate, and 6 grams fat

*Chicken Avocado Spinach Salad

Salad:

Mixed greens

4 ounces cooked chicken

2 tablespoons sunflower
  seeds

1 tablespoon dried cranberries

¼ avocado, pitted, peeled, and
  sliced

Dressing:

1 tablespoon freshly squeezed
  lemon juice

1 garlic clove, minced

1 teaspoon Dijon mustard

1 teaspoon avocado oil

Place the mixed greens on a plate. Top with the chicken, sunflower seeds, cranberries, and avocado. Whisk together the dressing ingredients in a small bowl. Drizzle over the salad.

Nutrition: 377 calories, 33 grams protein, 15 grams carbohydrate, and 21 grams fat

Guacamole Chicken Salad

5 ounces grilled or roasted
  chicken, shredded

¼ cup mashed avocado

1 cup greens (spinach, kale, or
  mixed)

2 tablespoons pico de gallo or
  salsa

In a small bowl, mix the chicken and avocado so that the avocado coats the chicken. Serve over the greens and top with pico de gallo.

Nutrition: 292 calories, 37 grams protein, 9 grams carbohydrate, and 13 grams fat

*Chicken Kale Salad and Lemon Vinaigrette

Salad:

2 cups baby kale

4 ounces grilled chicken

½ cup cored and chopped
   apple

1 ounce raw almonds

Vinaigrette:

1 teaspoon olive oil

2 tablespoons freshly
   squeezed lemon juice

Assemble the salad: Place the kale on a plate.
Add the chicken, apple, and almonds.

Make the vinaigrette: In a small bowl, whisk
together the oil and lemon juice. Drizzle over
the salad.

*Nutrition: 355 calories, 37 grams protein, 26 grams carbohydrate, and
16 grams fat*

*Apple Walnut Chicken Salad

2 cups organic kale

4 ounces cooked chicken
   breast

¼ apple, cored and chopped

⅛ cup walnuts

2 tablespoons goat cheese

1 teaspoon grapeseed oil

Place the kale on a plate. In a small bowl, toss
together the remaining ingredients. Serve
over the kale.

*Nutrition: 441 calories, 39 grams protein, 25 grams carbohydrate, and
54 grams fat*

Turkey and Sweet Potato Casserole

Vegetable oil spray
4 ounces lean ground turkey
4 ounces baked sweet potato,
   cut into cubes
½ cup egg whites
½ cup seeded and chopped
   green and red bell pepper

Preheat the oven to 325°F. Spray a small baking dish with vegetable oil.

In a small bowl, combine all the remaining ingredients. Mix well. Transfer to the prepared baking dish. Bake for 30 to 40 minutes, or until cooked through.

Nutrition: 307 calories, 36 grams protein, 25 grams carbohydrate, and 8 grams fat

*Lean Turkey Dinner

Vegetable oil spray
1 (6-ounce) lean turkey patty
1 (4-ounce) sweet potato,
   baked
1 cup steamed broccoli

Spray a small skillet with vegetable oil.

Over medium-high heat, pan-fry the turkey patty on both sides in the prepared skillet until cooked throughout.

Scoop out the baked sweet potato flesh and mash well. Serve with the broccoli.

Nutrition: 394 calories, 38 grams protein, 36 grams carbohydrate, and 12 grams fat

*Protein-Packed Cauliflower Mash

Vegetable oil spray
5 ounces lean ground turkey
1 cup mashed cauliflower,
  prepared from frozen
2 tablespoons salsa
¼ avocado, peeled and sliced

Spray a small skillet coated with vegetable oil spray. In the prepared skillet, brown the turkey over medium-high heat. Stir in the cauliflower. Serve, topped with the salsa and avocado.

Nutrition: 320 calories, 32 grams protein, 21 grams carbohydrate, and 15 grams fat

Turkey Slider with Sweet Potato Bun

6 ounces sweet potato
3 ounces lean ground turkey
2 teaspoons Dijon mustard
2 tablespoons shredded
  mozzarella cheese
2 tomato slices
A few spinach leaves
Salt and freshly ground black
  pepper

Preheat the oven to 375°F.

Peel and then cut the sweet potato into four rounds. Please on a baking sheet and bake for 40 to 45 minutes, or until soft.

Form the turkey into two small patties. Grill or pan-fry over medium heat until cooked through.

Spread the potato rounds with mustard. Place the turkey, cheese, tomato slices, and spinach between the rounds to create "sliders."

Nutrition: 290 calories, 25 grams protein, 36 grams carbohydrate, and 3 grams fat

Ezekiel Turkey Sandwich

2 teaspoons honey mustard
2 slices Ezekiel bread
4 ounces Applegate Farms
   sliced turkey or other
   deli-type turkey
1 tomato slice

Spread the honey mustard on the bread slices. Sandwich the turkey and tomato between the bread.

Nutrition: 282 calories, 32 grams protein, 31 grams carbohydrate, and 3 grams fat

Pork Tenderloin and Roasted Potatoes

Marinade:
1 teaspoon Worcestershire
   sauce
1 tablespoon organic ketchup
1 teaspoon chili powder
1 teaspoon cider vinegar
1 teaspoon pure maple syrup

4 ounces pork tenderloin
1 cup quartered red-skinned
   potatoes
1 tablespoon olive oil

In a small bowl, whisk together the marinade ingredients.

Place the pork in the bowl and marinate in the refrigerator at least 2 hours, or overnight.

Preheat the oven to 350°F.

Place the potatoes and oil in a resealable plastic bag to let the oil coat the potatoes.

Roast the pork in a small baking dish for at least 20 minutes.

Place the oil-coated potatoes in the baking dish and roast alongside the pork until the potatoes are tender, about 30 minutes.

Nutrition: 349 calories, 34 grams protein, 41 grams carbohydrate, and 4 grams fat

Buffalo Chicken Meatballs

Makes 24 meatballs (6 meatballs = 1 serving)

1¼ pounds ground chicken
¼ cup whole wheat panko
   bread crumbs
1 large egg
2 chopped scallions
⅓ cup minced celery
⅓ cup grated carrot
1 garlic clove, minced
⅓ cup Frank's RedHot sauce
Salt and freshly ground black
   pepper

Preheat the oven to 400°F.

In a large bowl, combine all the ingredients and form into two dozen equal-size balls. Place on a baking sheet and bake until browned and cooked through, about 30 minutes.

Nutrition: 264 calories, 29 grams protein, 4 grams carbohydrate, and 14 grams fat

*Coconut-Crusted Chicken Fingers

Vegetable oil spray
¼ cup unsweetened coconut
   flakes
⅛ cup finely chopped almonds
4 ounces chicken tenders
¼ cup egg whites, slightly
   beaten

Preheat the oven to 425°F. Spray a baking dish with vegetable oil.

In a shallow bowl, combine the coconut flakes and almonds.

Dip each tender into the egg whites, then roll in the coconut mixture to fully coat the tenders.

Place the tenders on the prepared baking dish. Bake until crispy and cooked throughout, about 30 minutes. Serve with a steamed vegetable side dish or baked sweet potato.

Nutrition: 270 calories, 39 grams protein, 7 grams carbohydrate, and 19 grams fat

*Stuffed 'Bellos

5 ounces shredded cooked
   chicken
½ cup chopped steamed or
   boiled brussels sprouts
1 teaspoon olive oil
1 teaspoon balsamic vinegar
Salt and freshly ground
   pepper
1 portobello mushroom cap,
   grilled or broiled

In a medium-size bowl, combine the chicken, brussels sprouts, oil, vinegar, and seasonings. Place atop the mushroom. Reheat if necessary.

Nutrition: 320 calories, 48 grams protein, 9 grams carbohydrate, and 10 grams fat

*Chicken Fajita Bowl

1 tablespoon olive oil
½ cup chopped onion
½ cup seeded and chopped
   bell pepper
¼ cup cooked brown rice
2 ounces cooked and
   shredded chicken
2 tablespoons black beans
2 tablespoons salsa
1 tablespoon shredded
   Cheddar cheese
1 tablespoon plain fat-free
   Greek yogurt

In a small skillet, heat the olive oil over medium heat and sauté the onion and pepper until tender. Remove from the heat and set aside.

In a serving bowl, layer the rice, chicken, onion, pepper, and black beans. Top with the salsa, cheese, and yogurt.

Nutrition: 292 calories, 26 grams protein, 38 grams carbohydrate, and 6 grams fat

Creamy Cauliflower Soup

1 tablespoon olive oil

2 cups chopped cauliflower

¼ cup chopped onion

1 garlic clove, minced

1 cup chicken broth

½ cup plain fat-free Greek
yogurt

2 ounces shredded cooked
chicken

⅓ cup shredded mozzarella
cheese

Heat the olive oil over medium heat. Sauté the cauliflower, onion, and garlic until soft. Transfer to a blender. Add the chicken broth and yogurt. Blend until creamy.

Place the mixture in a medium saucepan and heat over medium heat. Pour into a soup bowl and top with the chicken and cheese.

Nutrition: 28 calories, 33 grams protein, 16 grams carbohydrate, and 11 grams fat

Open-Faced Tuna Sandwich

4 ounces wild-caught tuna

1 cup spinach, chopped

1 teaspoon grapeseed oil

1 slice Ezekiel bread

In a small bowl, toss the tuna with spinach and oil. Lightly toast the bread. Top the bread with the tuna mixture and serve.

Nutrition: 272 calories, 32 grams protein, 16 grams carbohydrate, and 9 grams fat

*Mustard Salmon with Grilled Asparagus

1 tablespoon Dijon mustard
1 garlic clove, minced
Juice of ½ lemon
5 ounces wild salmon
12 asparagus spears, grilled

Preheat the oven to 400°F.

In a small bowl, whisk together the mustard, garlic, and lemon juice. Place the salmon in a small glass baking dish. Pour the mustard mixture over the fish. Bake for 10 to 12 minutes, or until the salmon flakes easily with a fork. Serve with the grilled asparagus.

Nutrition: 326 calories, 42 grams protein, 11 grams carbohydrate, and 12 grams fat

Smoked Salmon Roll-Ups

1 (4-ounce) package smoked
  salmon
1 small avocado, pitted,
  peeled, and mashed

Place the salmon on a plate. Spread with the mashed avocado. Roll up and slice into pinwheels. Serve with a side salad.

Nutrition: 212 calories, 22 grams protein, 4 grams carbohydrate, and 12 grams fat

Citrus Fish Tacos

4 ounces grilled white fish, such as mahi-mahi tilapia, or halibut, cut into small chunks

½ small avocado, pitted, peeled, and sliced

1 tablespoon plain fat-free Greek yogurt

½ Roma tomato, diced

1 tablespoon chopped fresh cilantro

2 butter lettuce cups

In a medium bowl, mix the fish, avocado, yogurt, tomato, and cilantro.

Make the vinaigrette: In a small bowl, whisk together the vinaigrette ingredients. Add the vinaigrette to the fish mixture and toss well.

Divide the mixture between the lettuce cups and serve.

Vinaigrette:

1 tablespoon freshly squeezed lime juice

1 tablespoon cider vinegar

½ teaspoon onion powder

Nutrition: 265 calories, 25 grams protein, 18 grams carbohydrate, and 12 grams fat

*Bison and Sweet Potato Mash

6 ounces ground bison

1 medium-size sweet potato, baked

Form the meat into a patty. Pan-fry in a small skillet over medium heat to your desired doneness. Scoop out the sweet potato flesh and mash. Serve together.

Nutrition: 498 calories, 42 grams protein, 23 grams carbohydrate, and 26 grams fat

Bunless Burger

5 ounces lean ground beef

½ cup cooked spinach

4 pieces sun-dried tomato, drained

Large lettuce leaf

Form the beef into a patty. Pan-fry in a small skillet over medium heat until cooked as desired.

Top the hamburger with the spinach and tomato. Wrap in the large lettuce leaf.

Nutrition: 245 calories, 31 grams protein, 3.5 grams carbohydrate, and 12 grams fat

Takeout-Style Beef and Mixed Veggies

Vegetable oil spray

4 ounces London broil, sliced, or flank steak strips

1 cup chopped broccoli

1 cup seeded and chopped red bell pepper

2 tablespoons coconut aminos

Cauliflower rice, cooked (optional)

Spray a small skillet with vegetable oil. In the prepared skillet, brown the meat over medium heat. Add the vegetables and coconut aminos. Cook until the veggies are crisp-tender, 6 to 8 minutes. Serve with cauliflower rice (if using).

Nutrition: 249 calories, 20 grams protein, 21 grams carbohydrate, and 5 grams fat

*Beef and Quinoa Naked Burrito

Vegetable oil spray
3 ounces grass-fed
  ground beef
½ cup cooked quinoa
¼ cup chopped onion
¼ cup seeded chopped bell
  pepper
1 teaspoon taco seasoning

Spray a small skillet with vegetable oil. In the prepared skillet, brown the meat over medium heat. Add the remaining ingredients and cook until the vegetables are soft.

Nutrition: 315 calories, 22 grams protein, 28 grams carbohydrate, and 13 grams fat

SMOOTHIES, SNACKS, AND DESSERTS

*Mint Milkshake

1½ cups unsweetened vanilla
  almond milk
2 Medjool dates, pitted
1 tablespoon cashew or
  almond butter
1 scoop Afterburn vanilla
  protein powder or other
  vanilla protein powder
1 capful mint extract
Handful of crushed ice

Place all the ingredients in a blender and blend until smooth.

Nutrition: 369 calories, 28 grams protein, 41 grams carbohydrate, and 13 grams fat

Piña Colada Smoothie

½ cup plain fat-free Greek
   yogurt
¾ cup unsweetened
   coconut milk
½ frozen banana
½ cup crushed pineapple in its
   own juice, drained
½ teaspoon coconut extract
2 teaspoons honey

Place all the ingredients in a blender and blend until smooth.

Nutrition: 274 calories, 14 grams protein, 40 grams carbohydrate, and 7.5 grams fat

Fruit and Veggie Shake

1½ cups unsweetened
   almond milk
½ cup frozen unsweetened
   mixed fruit
½ frozen banana
Handful of fresh spinach
   or kale
1 scoop Afterburn vanilla
   protein powder or other
   vanilla protein powder

Place all the ingredients in a blender and blend until smooth.

Nutrition: 270 calories, 28 grams protein, 33 grams carbohydrate, and 5 grams fat

*Chocolate Banana Smoothie

1 cup unsweetened
almond milk
1 scoop Afterburn chocolate
protein powder or other
chocolate protein powder
1 tablespoon almond butter
1 medium-size ripe banana

Place all the ingredients in a blender and blend until smooth.

Nutrition: 341 calories, 28 grams protein, 33 grams carbohydrate, and 14 grams fat

*Afterburn Coffee

1 cup brewed coffee, at room
temperature
½ cup unsweetened
almond milk
1 scoop Afterburn protein
powder
¼ teaspoon ground cinnamon
1½ teaspoons coconut oil
6 to 8 ice cubes

Place all the ingredients in a blender and blend until smooth.

Nutrition: 192 calories, 24 grams protein, 6 grams carbohydrate, and 10 grams fat

*Protein Power Cups

Vegetable oil spray
¼ cup egg whites
1 ounce ground turkey
¼ cup seeded and chopped
  bell pepper
1 tablespoon goat cheese

Preheat the oven to 375°F. Spray one or two muffin cups with vegetable oil.

In a small bowl, combine all the ingredients and mix well. Transfer to the prepared muffin cup(s). Bake for 30 minutes.

Nutrition: 100 calories, 16 grams protein, 2 grams carbohydrate, and 16 grams fat

Pesto Cauliflower

1 cup steamed or roasted
  cauliflower pieces
1 tablespoon pesto sauce

In a small bowl, coat the cauliflower with the pesto sauce and serve.

Nutrition: 82 calories, 3 grams protein, 6 grams carbohydrate, and 6 grams fat

*Protein Brownie Mug Cake

¼ cup unsweetened
  almond milk
1 scoop Afterburn protein
  powder or other protein
  powder
1½ teaspoons unsweetened
  cocoa powder
½ tablespoon coconut flour
½ teaspoon baking powder
5 to 10 drops liquid stevia

Combine all the ingredients in a microwave-safe mug. Mix well. Microwave on HIGH for 20 to 30 seconds.

Nutrition: 190 calories, 27 grams protein, 15 grams carbohydrate, and 4 grams fat

*Chocolate Chip Cookie Dough Pudding

6 ounces plain fat-free Greek
  yogurt
½ banana, mashed
1 tablespoon powdered
  peanut butter
½ scoop Afterburn protein
  powder or other protein
  powder
1 tablespoon
  stevia-sweetened chocolate
  chips, such as Lily's

In a small bowl, mix all the ingredients. Chill for at least 1 hour, then serve.

Nutrition: 239 calories, 30 grams protein, 28 grams carbohydrate, and 5 grams fat

*Apples and Peanut Butter

3 tablespoons plain fat-free
  Greek yogurt
½ scoop Afterburn protein
  powder or other protein
  powder
2 tablespoons powdered
  peanut butter
Pinch of ground cinnamon
1 small apple, cored and sliced

In a small bowl, whisk together the yogurt, protein power, peanut butter, and cinnamon. Spread the mixture over the apple slices and enjoy.

Nutrition: 202 calories, 21 grams protein, 30 grams carbohydrate, and 2 grams fat

REFERENCES

PART 1: INNER AND OUTER TRANSFORMATION

Chapter 1—Strategy #1: Burn

Čukić, I. "Childhood IQ and Survival to 79: Follow-Up of 94% of the Scottish Mental Survey 1947." *Intelligence* 63 (2017): 45–50.

Daniel, J. Z., et al. "The Effect of Exercise in Reducing Desire to Smoke and Cigarette Withdrawal Symptoms Is Not Caused by Distraction." *Addiction* 101, no. 8 (2006): 1187–1192.

Dunton, G. F., et al. "Momentary Assessment of Contextual Influences on Affective Response During Physical Activity." *Health Psychology* 34, no. 12 (2015): 1145–1153.

Morales, J. I. "The Heart's Electromagnetic Field Is Your Superpower: Training Heart-Brain Coherence." *Psychology Today*, November 29, 2020. https://www.psychology today.com/us/blog/building-the-habit-of-hero/202011/the-hearts-electromagnetic -field-is-your-superpower.

Rassovsky, Y., et al. "Martial Arts Increase Oxytocin Production." *Scientific Reports* 9, no. 1 (2019): 12980.

Singh, B., et al. "Effectiveness of Physical Activity Interventions for Improving Depression, Anxiety and Distress: An Overview of Systematic Reviews." *British Journal of Sports Medicine*, February 16, 2023. https://pubmed.ncbi.nlm.nih.gov/36796860/.

Chapter 2—Strategy #2: Believe

Carver, C. S., et al. "Optimism." *Clinical Psychology Review* 30, no. 7 (2010): 879–889.

Kato, K., et al. "Positive Attitude Towards Life, Emotional Expression, Self-Rated Health, and Depressive Symptoms Among Centenarians and Near-Centenarians." *Aging & Mental Health* 20, no. 9 (2016): 930–939.

Krittanawong, C., et al. "Association of Pessimism with Cardiovascular Events and All-Cause Mortality." *Progress in Cardiovascular Diseases* 76 (2023): 91–98.

Seligman, M. E. P., *Learned Optimism—How to Change Your Mind and Your Life.* (New York: Random House, 2006), 4–5.

Chapter 3—Strategy #3: Nourish

Boushey, C., et al. "Dietary Patterns and Neurocognitive Health: A Systematic Review." US Department of Agriculture, Nutrition Evidence Systematic Review, July 2020. https://pubmed.ncbi.nlm.nih.gov/35129905/.

Halvorson, H. G. "The 2 Words You Have to Stop Saying (or Thinking) Today." *Psychology Today*, January 18, 2018. https://www.psychologytoday.com/us/blog/the-science-of-success/201301/the-2-words-you-have-to-stop-saying-or-thinking-today.

Hulsken, S., et al. "Food-Derived Serotonergic Modulators: Effects on Mood and Cognition." *Nutrition Research Reviews* 26 (2013): 223–234.

Jacka, F. N., et al. "Association of Western and Traditional Diets with Depression and Anxiety in Women." *American Journal of Psychiatry* 167, no. 3 (2010): 305–311.

Rahman, M., and A. B. Berenson. "Self-Perception of Weight and Its Association with Weight-Related Behaviors in Young, Reproductive-Aged Women." *Obstetrics and Gynecology* 116, no. 6 (2010): 1274–1280.

Shin, J. H. "Consumption of 85% Cocoa Dark Chocolate Improves Mood in Association with Gut Microbial Changes in Healthy Adults: A Randomized Controlled Trial." *Journal of Nutritional Biochemistry* 99, no. 6 (2020): 108854.

Yılmaz, C., and V. Gökmen. "Neuroactive Compounds in Foods: Occurrence, Mechanism and Potential Health Effects." *Food Research International* 128, no. 3 (2020): 108744.

Chapter 4—Strategy #4: Achieve

Aron, A., et al. "Reward, Motivation, and Emotion Systems Associated with Early-Stage Intense Romantic Love." *Journal of Neurophysiology* 94, no. 1 (2005): 327–337.

Shilts, M. K., et al. "Goal Setting as a Strategy for Dietary and Physical Activity Behavior Change: A Review of the Literature." *American Journal of Health Promotion* 19, no. 2 (2004): 81–93.

Chapter 5—Strategy #5: Connect

Berkman, L. F., and S. L. Syme. "Social Networks, Host Resistance, and Mortality: A Nine-Year Follow-Up Study of Alameda County Residents." *American Journal of Epidemiology* 109, no. 2 (1979): 186–204.

Cohen-Cole, E., and J. M. Fletcher. "Is Obesity Contagious? Social Networks vs. Environmental Factors in the Obesity Epidemic." *Journal of Health Economics* 27, no. 5 (2008): 1382–1387.

Cole, S. W., et al. "Myeloid Differentiation Architecture of Leukocyte Transcriptome Dynamics in Perceived Social Isolation." *Proceedings of the National Academy of Sciences* 112, no. 49 (2015): 15142–15147.

Hill, A. L., et al. "Infectious Disease Modeling of Social Contagion in Networks." *PLoS Computational Biology* 6, no. 11 (2010): e1000968.

Holt-Lunstad, J. "Why Social Relationships Are Important for Physical Health: A Systems Approach to Understanding and Modifying Risk and Protection." *Annual Review of Psychology* 69 (2018): 437–458.

Jackson, S. E., et al. "The Influence of Partner's Behavior on Health Behavior Change: The English Longitudinal Study of Ageing." *JAMA Internal Medicine* 175, no 3 (2015): 385–392.

Martino, J., et al. "The Connection Prescription: Using the Power of Social Interactions and the Deep Desire for Connectedness to Empower Health and Wellness." *American Journal of Lifestyle Medicine* 11, no. 6 (2015): 466–475.

Rutledge, T., et al. "Social Networks Are Associated with Lower Mortality Rates Among Women with Suspected Coronary Disease: The National Heart, Lung, and Blood Institute-Sponsored Women's Ischemia Syndrome Evaluation Study." *Psychosomatic Medicine* 66, no. 6 (2004): 882–888.

PART 2: CREATE THE LIFE YOU LOVE

Chapter 6—Let's Get Moving

Archila, L. R., et al. "Simple Bodyweight Training Improves Cardiorespiratory Fitness with Minimal Time Commitment: A Contemporary Application of the 5BX Approach." *International Journal of Exercise Science* 14, no. 3 (2021): 93–100.

Krzysztof, L., et al. "The Impact of Ten Weeks of Bodyweight Training on the Level of Physical Fitness and Selected Parameters of Body Composition in Women Aged 21–23 Years." *Polish Journal of Sport and Tourism* 22, no. 2 (2015): 64–68.

Myers, T. R., et al. "Whole-Body Aerobic Resistance Training Circuit Improves Aerobic Fitness and Muscle Strength in Sedentary Young Females." *Journal of the Strength and Conditioning Association* 29, no. 6 (2015): 1592–1600.

Yang, J., et al. "Association Between Push-Up Exercise Capacity and Future Cardiovascular Events Among Active Adult Men." *JAMA Network Open* 2, no. 2 (2019): e188341.

Chapter 7—What You Think, You Create

Hill, P. L., and N. A. Turiano. "Purpose in Life as a Predictor of Mortality Across Adulthood." *Psychological Science* 25, no. 7 (2014): 1482–1486.

Lester, D., et al. "Maslow's Hierarchy of Needs and Psychological Health." *Journal of General Psychology* 109, no. 1 (1983): 83–85.

Tod, D., et al. "Effects of Self-Talk: A Systematic Review." *Journal of Sport & Exercise Psychology* 33, no. 5 (2011): 666–687.

Chapter 8—Nutrition Is Critical, but Easier Than You Think

Antonio, J. "High-Protein Diets in Trained Individuals." *Research in Sports Medicine* 27, no. 2 (2019): 195–203.

Yi, S. Y., et al. "Added Sugar Intake Is Associated with Pericardial Adipose Tissue." *European Journal of Preventive Cardiology* 27 (2020): 2016–2023.

Chapter 9—Achieve What Your Heart Desires

Abdulla, A., et al. "Guidance on the Management of Pain in Older People." *Age and Ageing* 42, suppl. 1 (2013): 1–57.

Huang, S. C., et al. "So Near and Yet So Far: The Mental Representation of Goal Progress." *Journal of Personality and Social Psychology* 103, no. 2 (2012): 225–241.

Mastropieri, B., et al. "Inner Resources for Survival: Integrating Interpersonal Psychotherapy with Spiritual Visualization with Homeless Youth." *Journal of Religion and Health* 54, no. 3 (2015): 903–921.

Ranganathan, V. K., et al. "From Mental Power to Muscle Power—Gaining Strength by Using the Mind." *Neuropsychologia* 42, no. 7 (2004): 944–956.

Chapter 10—Create Your Circle of Connection

Beamish, A, J., et al. "What's in a Smile? A Review of the Benefits of the Clinician's Smile." *Postgraduate Medical Journal* 95, no. 1120 (2019): 91–95.

Dunbar, R. I. M. "The Anatomy of Friendship." *Trends in Cognitive Sciences* 22, no. 1 (2018): 32–51.

Guiney, H., and L. Machado. "Volunteering in the Community: Potential Benefits for Cognitive Aging." *Journals of Gerontology* 73, no. 3 (2018): 399–408.

Holt-Lunstad, J. "Why Social Relationships Are Important for Physical Health: A Systems Approach to Understanding and Modifying Risk and Protection." *Annual Review of Psychology* 69 (2018): 437–445.

Martino, J., et al. "The Connection Prescription: Using the Power of Social Interactions and the Deep Desire for Connectedness to Empower Health and Wellness." *American Journal of Lifestyle Medicine* 11, no. 6 (2015): 466–475.

McCoy, L. A. "The Power of Your Vocal Image." *Journal of the Canadian Dental Association* 62, no. 3 (1996): 231–234.

von Bonsdorff, M. B., and T. Rantanen. "Benefits of Formal Voluntary Work Among Older People. A Review." *Aging Clinical and Experimental Research* 23, no. 3 (2011): 162–169.

ACKNOWLEDGMENTS

On our two-year journey of crafting *Burn*, so many hands and hearts have contributed to this life-changing project. The gratitude we feel is profound and infinite.

To our members featured in this book: Cynthia Russe, Hope Gibson, Kellie Sprouse, Eliza Peterson, Karen Borgrud, Tori Villarreal, Elaine Tylus, Samantha Rey, Brian Woddell, Tiffany Yager, Jessie Winnie, Drew Ford, Gaige Kartchner, and Kifa Johnston—thank you. Your honesty and example will inspire the world.

To our franchise partners: You have amplified our message, allowing us to reach countless hearts. The strategies on these pages reflect the life-changing mission we have all dedicated ourselves to, and we could not do this without your love and support.

To our team members: Every day, you wake up early and stay up late to serve your community. You embody the spirit of *Burn*, both within the pages of this book and beyond. You are the heartbeat to our community.

And to those special mentions who helped *Burn* come to life: Matt Morris, Ansley Melnik, Isaiah Hammond, DJ Splain, Trish Pena, and the team at Burn HQ. We are proud of you beyond belief.

We would like to thank our agent, Tom Miller, for his editorial guidance and for coordinating with our publisher, Hachette Go. We are grateful to our collaborator Maggie Greenwood-Robinson for her exceptional research skills, her help with the organization of our manuscript, and her editorial creativity in helping bring to life the book we envisioned.

Thanks also to Dan Ambrosio, Michael Barrs, Kindall Gant, and Michelle Aielli at Hachette Go, and to Kevin Anderson, for his initial help.

To everyone who's interacted with us in the gym or online—you've played a part in this journey, and we're thankful every day we get to serve you and your family. Every word on these pages represents you: true believers. We never take your trust in us for granted and have dedicated our lives to the mission.

Your belief in us is the fuel to our fire. Together, we can go much further than we can alone.

INDEX

accountability
  for achieving goals, 1–2, 89–90,
    100–102
  calorie accountability, 66–69, 150–151,
    153–154
  commitment and, 89–90, 100–102
  community and, 89–91, 101
  connections and, 89–90, 126
Achieve strategy
  explanation of, 12, 73–76
  North Star goals, 74–83, 87–89, 137,
    171–181, 198–200
  reviewing, 198
  "small wins," 77–78, 170–171, 175
Addiction (journal), 23
addictions
  alcoholism, 6–7, 21, 24–25, 37–39, 150
  cigarettes, 21–23
  drug addiction, 21–22
  exercise and, 21–24
  "positive addiction," 23
  withdrawal symptoms, 23–25
  workouts and, 21–24
adrenaline, 27
afterburn effect, 111
alcohol consumption, 6–7, 21–25, 37–39,
    88, 99, 150, 167, 176, 184
alcoholism, 6–7, 21, 24–25, 37–39, 150
Alzheimer's disease, 28
American Psychiatric Association, 20
anchors, 10, 31, 72, 101, 141
antidepressants, 19–20, 183
anxiety

impact of, 3–4, 7, 39
reducing, 4, 10–11, 19–20, 28, 59, 92–94,
  172, 177
self-limiting beliefs and, 135–136
universal needs and, 139–140
appetite, controlling, 58, 64–65, 149
appetite suppressants, 9, 61, 146
apps, 67, 101–102, 154, 190–191
Atleto, 191
attitude
  beliefs and, 39–50, 134–138, 198
  changing, 47–50, 134–135, 198
  effort and, 44, 47–50, 134–135
  explanation of, 47–48
  failure and, 40, 43–48, 65, 73–74, 134
  goals and, 39–50, 83, 174, 197–200
  importance of, 39–50
  negative attitude, 43, 47–50
  positive attitude, 39–50, 83, 133–136,
    183–184, 197–200
  success and, 40–50, 73–74, 134

bad habits, breaking, 13, 21–24, 88, 141,
    151–152, 186
Battle Creek, Michigan, 8, 127
beliefs
  attitude and, 39–50, 134–138, 198
  belief systems, 40–52, 140–143, 198
  changing, 39–52, 134–135, 198
  connections and, 42, 50–52
  effort and, 44, 47–50
  importance of, 6, 40–52
  inner strength and, 11, 40–52